Allergy and Immunology

Editors

ANDREW LUTZKANIN III
KRISTEN M. LUTZKANIN

PRIMARY CARE:
CLINICS IN OFFICE PRACTICE

www.primarycare.theclinics.com

Consulting Editor
JOEL J. HEIDELBAUGH

June 2023 • Volume 50 • Number 2

ELSEVIER

1600 John F. Kennedy Boulevard ● Suite 1800 ● Philadelphia, Pennsylvania, 19103-2899

http://www.theclinics.com

PRIMARY CARE: CLINICS IN OFFICE PRACTICE Volume 50, Number 2
June 2023 ISSN 0095-4543, ISBN-13: 978-0-323-93909-6

Editor: Taylor Hayes
Developmental Editor: Jessica Cañaberal

Primary Care: Clinics in Office Practice (ISSN: 0095-4543) is published quarterly by Elsevier Inc., 360 Park Avenue South, New York, NY 10010-1710. Months of issue are March, June, September, and December. Periodicals postage paid at New York, NY and additional mailing offices. Subscription prices are $277.00 per year (US individuals), $629.00 (US institutions), $100.00 (US students), $321.00 (Canadian individuals), $712.00 (Canadian institutions), $100.00 (Canadian students), $379.00 (international individuals), $712.00 (international institutions), and $175.00 (international students). Foreign air speed delivery is included in all *Clinics* subscription prices. All prices are subject to change without notice. POSTMASTER: Send address changes to *Primary Care: Clinics in Office Practice*, Elsevier Periodicals Customer Service, 11830 Westline Industrial Drive, St. Louis, MO 63146. Customer Service Health Sciences Division, Subscription Customer Service, 3251 Riverport Lane, Maryland Heights, MO 63043. **Customer Service: 1-800-654-2452 (U.S. and Canada); 314-447-8871 (outside U.S. and Canada). Fax: 314-447-8029. E-mail: journalscustomerservice-usa@elsevier.com (for print support); journalsonlinesupport-usa@elsevier.com (for online support).**

Reprints. For copies of 100 or more, of articles in this publication, please contact the Commercial Reprints Department, Elsevier Inc., 360 Park Avenue South, New York, NY 10010-1710. Tel. 212-633-3874; Fax: 212-633-3820; E-mail: reprints@elsevier.com.

Primary Care: Clinics in Office Practice is covered in *MEDLINE/PubMed (Index Medicus)* and *EMBASE/Excerpta Medica, Current Contents/Clinical Medicine, and ISI/BIOMED.*

Contributors

CONSULTING EDITOR

JOEL J. HEIDELBAUGH, MD, FAAFP, FACG
Clinical Professor, Departments of Family Medicine and Urology, Director of Medical Student Education and Clerkship Director, Department of Family Medicine, University of Michigan Medical School, Ann Arbor, Michigan; Ypsilanti Health Center, Ypsilanti, Michigan

EDITORS

ANDREW LUTZKANIN III, MD, FAAFP
Associate Professor, Department of Family and Community Medicine, Penn State College of Medicine, Hershey, Pennsylvania

KRISTEN M. LUTZKANIN, MD
Assistant Professor, Department of Pediatrics, Penn State College of Medicine, Hershey, Pennsylvania

AUTHORS

DOERTHE A. ANDREAE, MD, PhD
Associate Professor, Division of Allergy and Immunology, Department of Dermatology, University of Utah, Salt Lake City, Utah

CAROLYN H. BALOH, MD
Division of Allergy and Clinical Immunology, Department of Medicine, Harvard Medical School, Brigham and Women's Hospital, Boston, Massachusetts

HEY CHONG, MD, PhD
Division of Allergy and Immunology, Department of Pediatrics, UPMC Children's Hospital of Pittsburgh, Pittsburgh, Pennsylvania

KARL T. CLEBAK, MD, MHA, FAAFP
Program Director, Associate Professor, Department of Family and Community Medicine, Penn State Health Milton. S Hershey Medical Center, Hershey, Pennsylvania

TIMOTHY CRAIG, DO
Professor of Medicine, Pediatrics and Biomedical Sciences, Penn State University, Hershey, Pennsylvania

ERIC J. CZECH, MSBS, PA-C
Assistant Professor, Division of Physician Assistant Studies, Department of Family Medicine, The University of Toledo College of Medicine and Life Sciences, Toledo, Ohio

CHRISTOPHER R. DAVIS, MD, MPH
Assistant Professor, Department of Family and Community Medicine, Penn State Health
Milton. S Hershey Medical Center, Hershey, Pennsylvania

KELAN FOGARTY, BS
Pennsylvania State University, College of Medicine University Park, Penn State College of
Medicine, State College, Pennsylvania

ESTELLE A. GREEN, BS
Pennsylvania State University, College of Medicine University Park, Penn State College of
Medicine, State College, Pennsylvania

LEESHA HELM, MD, MPH
Assistant Professor, Department of Family and Community Medicine, Penn State Health
Milton. S Hershey Medical Center, Hershey, Pennsylvania

MATTHEW F. HELM, MD
Assistant Professor, Department of Dermatology, Penn State Health Milton. S Hershey
Medical Center, Hershey, Pennsylvania

ALEXANDRA HORWITZ, MD, FAAAAI
Associate Professor of Pediatrics and Medicine, Division of Allergy-Immunology, Penn
State Health Children's Hospital, Hershey, Pennsylvania

FAOUD T. ISHMAEL, MD, PhD
Pennsylvania State University, College of Medicine University Park, Mount Nittany Health,
State College, Pennsylvania

CHELSEA ELIZABETH MENDONCA, MD
Chief Resident, Department of Family and Community Medicine, Baylor College of
Medicine, Houston, Texas

SARAH MERRILL, MD
Assistant Professor of Family Medicine and Public Health, Family Medicine Department,
UC San Diego Health, San Diego, California

MUNIMA NASIR, MD, FAAFP
Associate Professor, Family and Community Medicine, Penn State Health Milton S.
Hershey Medical Center, Hershey, Pennsylvania

HUONG NGUYEN, DO, MS
Resident Physician, Family and Community Medicine, Penn State Health Milton S.
Hershey Medical Center, Hershey, Pennsylvania

CRYSTAL NWAGWU, MD
Assistant Professor, Department of Family and Community Medicine, Baylor College of
Medicine, Houston, Texas

ANDREW OVERHOLSER, MSBS, PA-C
Assistant Professor, Division of Physician Assistant Studies, Department of Family
Medicine, The University of Toledo College of Medicine and Life Sciences, Toledo, Ohio

ARINDAM SARKAR, MD
Assistant Professor, Department of Family and Community Medicine, Baylor College of
Medicine, Houston, Texas

PAUL SCHAEFER, MD, PhD
Associate Professor, Department of Family Medicine, College of Medicine and Life Sciences, University of Toledo Medical Center, Toledo, Ohio

PAUL SCHULTZ, MD
Assistant Professor, Residency Program Director, Department of Family Medicine, The University of Toledo College of Medicine and Life Sciences, Toledo, Ohio

KATE SZYMANSKI, DO
Assistant Professor, Department of Family Medicine, College of Medicine and Life Sciences, University of Toledo Medical Center, Toledo, Ohio

KRISTA TODORIC, MD
Medical Arts Allergy, Carlisle, Pennsylvania

PRABHDEEP UPPAL, DO, MS
Resident Physician, Department of Family and Community Medicine, Department of Emergency Medicine, Wilmington, Delaware

BRIDGID WILSON, MD, PhD
Department of Community and Family Medicine, Assistant Professor, University Health Lakewood Medical Center, Kansas City, Missouri

J. LANE WILSON, MD, FAAFP
Department of Community and Family Medicine, Associate Professor, University of Missouri Kansas City School of Medicine, University Health Lakewood Medical Center, Kansas City, Missouri

SAMINA YUNUS, MD, MPH
Assistant Professor, Case Western Reserve School of Medicine, Staff Physician, Cleveland Clinic Department of Family Medicine, Chagrin Falls, Ohio

Contents

Allergic rhinitis is a common ailment in primary and acute care settings. Diagnosis is clinical, by means of history and physical examination. Referral to an allergist is considered when symptoms are difficult to manage and/or confirmation by means of further testing is desired. Management of allergic rhinitis should not be considered trivial, as multiple secondary effects can present as the course progresses. Several treatment modalities exist but should begin with glucocorticoid nasal sprays and systemic second- or third-generation antihistamines.

Asthma is characterized by chronic inflammation and respiratory symptoms such as wheezing and coughing. In the United States, it affects 25 million people annually. Chronic smokers, poor adherence to medications, incorrect use of inhalers, and overall poor asthma control are known risk factors that lead to poorly controlled chronic asthmatics. Although asthma is traditionally categorized by severity, treatment by primary care providers is guided by the Global Initiative for Asthma or the National Asthma Education and Prevention Program. As more research is available, shared decision-making between health care providers and patients will lead to improved outcomes in managing chronic asthma.

Atopic dermatitis (AD) is a common, chronic relapsing, and remitting inflammatory skin disease that is characterized by erythematous, scaly, and pruritic lesions often located over the flexural surfaces. Treatment goals of AD include the reduction of itching and burning, as well as the reduction of skin changes. Treatment of AD includes emollients and skin care, topical therapies including topical corticosteroids and steroid-sparing therapies, systemic therapies, and phototherapy.

from antibiotic prophylaxis to hematopoietic stem cell transplantation depending on the specific diagnosis.

Oral immunotherapy (OIT) is an alternative treatment of IgE-mediated food allergy that has been shown to increase tolerance threshold to many of the top food allergens, although this effect may be dependent on age, dose, frequency, and duration. OIT has been shown to be effective and safe in infants, and early initiation can improve rates of desensitization even for those foods whose natural history favors loss of allergy. Studies looking at protocol modification to improve OIT success are ongoing as is the evaluation of clinical tools to help monitor OIT effects.

This chapter presents an overview of eosinophilic esophagitis (EoE) for the Primary Care Practitioner (PCP). The focus is on helping PCPs keep it in their differential diagnosis by discussing the spectrum of clinical presentations, how to screen for EoE in at-risk populations and subsequently manage the patient with this condition. The authors review epidemiology, risk factors and associated conditions, pathology, clinical presentation, diagnosis, and management options.

Hereditary angioedema is a rare autosomal dominant condition characterized by episodes of swelling of the upper airway, intestines, and skin. The disorder is characterized by deficiency in C1 esterase inhibitor (C1-INH) or a decrease in functional C1-INH. Treatment options include on demand therapy (treatment of acute attacks), long-term prophylaxis, and short-term prophylaxis. Corticosteroids, epinephrine, and antihistamines are not effective for this form of angioedema. The high mortality in patients undiagnosed underscores a need for broader physician awareness to identify these patients and initiate therapy.

Stinging insects are a frequent cause of local and systemic hypersensitivity reactions, including anaphylaxis. For those with a history of life-threatening anaphylaxis, venom immunotherapy is effective, safe, and can be life-saving. Arachnids are a much less common source of envenomation through bites or stings and are less likely to cause a hypersensitivity reaction. However, recognizing the clinical manifestations when they do present is important for accurate diagnosis and treatment, and, when indicated, consideration of other diagnoses.

x

Allergy and Immunology
PRIMARY CARE:
CLINICS IN OFFICE PRACTICE

SERIES OF RELATED INTEREST

Medical Clinics (http://www.medical.theclinics.com)
Physician Assistant Clinics (https://www.physicianassistant.theclinics.com)

Foreword

Beeeeeee Careful

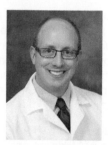

Joel J. Heidelbaugh, MD, FAAFP, FACG
Consulting Editor

The mystery of allergic conditions continues to expand and fascinate us. Theories abound regarding what is causing them, what is raising their incidence, and why they can occur later in life after assumed exposures. Is it changes in conventional farming and soil composition? Waning immunity? Altered pathogenicity of toxins? Randomness in the universe?

About a decade ago, I asked a colleague how his weekend was, and he replied, *"Great, until I almost died"*! Shocked, I asked him what happened, and he detailed how he had been stung by a bee when he was sitting on his porch. Within minutes, his hand swelled, then his arm, then his neck, and then his tongue. Fortunately, his wife (also a physician) was with him and made him immediately chew some Benadryl. They live within a few blocks of our University Hospital, and before the staff checked him in, the emergency department shot him with prednisone upon presentation and literally saved his life. Astonished by this story, I asked if he had ever been stung by a bee before, and he affirmed that he had dozens of stings throughout childhood when he frequently camped with his family. So why did this anaphylactic event occur now, so unpredictably? Always humorous, my colleague told me to *"Beeeeeeeeeee Careful"*!

This issue of *Primary Care: Clinics in Office Practice* highlights a collection of articles centered on the parent topic of allergy while providing current evidence and strategies on diagnosis and treatment. Our talented authors cover commonly encountered topics, including allergic rhinitis, chronic asthma, atopic dermatitis, urticaria, and angioedema. The article on inborn errors of immunity provides a solid basic science foundation for the general concepts across all of the articles within this issue. Food allergy is presented in a very logical fashion with salient information that can be readily used in an educational format during patient encounters. Admittedly, I never learned about eosinophilic esophagitis when I was in medical school in the 1990s, and much has been discovered about diagnostic and therapeutic strategies in the past decades. I

Prim Care Clin Office Pract 50 (2023) xi–xii
https://doi.org/10.1016/j.pop.2023.02.001
0095-4543/23/© 2023 Published by Elsevier Inc.

was very intrigued when I read the article on penicillin allergy since theoretically I have been allergic to penicillin since I was a young child. Now, new theories and strategies have raised the question of the validity of the persistence of such an allergy, and there are options to test and desensitize patients. Many clinicians reading this issue will learn the ground-breaking trend of oral immunotherapy, which has the potential for incorporation in primary care practices.

Drs Andrew and Kristen Lutzkanin have created a very unique collection of articles on the topic of allergy and many relative subtopics that we frequently encounter in our practices. As with every issue of *Primary Care: Clinics in Office Practice*, I not only self-ishly revel in refreshing my learned (and often forgotten) knowledge but also consider it the most cutting-edge form of continuing medical education. We hope that this issue will augment your comfort in diagnosing, treating, and preventing many common allergic conditions and syndromes in your respective practices.

Joel J. Heidelbaugh, MD, FAAFP, FACG
Departments of Family Medicine and Urology
Department of Family Medicine
University of Michigan Medical School
Ann Arbor, MI, USA

Ypsilanti Health Center
200 Arnet Suite 200
Ypsilanti, MI 48198, USA

E-mail address:
jheidel@umich.edu

Preface

Biologics, Single Maintenance and Reliever Therapy, Oral Immunotherapy, and More: Updates from the World of Allergy, Asthma, and Immunology

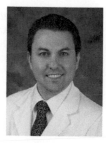 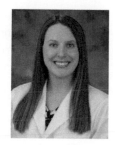

Andrew Lutzkanin III, MD, FAAFP   Kristen M. Lutzkanin, MD
Editors

Atopic conditions are common complaints in a primary care office. From atopic dermatitis to severe asthma and complicated food allergy, primary care physicians are the first stop for most allergic conditions. In the years since the first *Primary Care: Clinics in Office Practice* issue devoted to allergy-related disorders, there have been significant advancements in the treatment of atopic conditions with the development of biologics and the evolution of different types of immunotherapies, with a particular nod to advancements in oral immunotherapy for treatment of food allergy. These advancements inspired this new issue of *Primary Care: Clinics in Office Practice* focused on atopic conditions. In addition to updates on the management of commonly seen conditions, such as allergic rhinitis, chronic asthma, atopic dermatitis, and food allergy, we also include several new articles looking at inborn errors of immunity, oral immunotherapy, and hereditary angioedema. While many of the more advanced treatments discussed here may require consultation with a specialist for management, patients rely on the information provided by their well-trusted primary care provider to help them understand what a specialist may have to offer. Each article has been written to offer quick, evidence-based recommendations for clinical practice as well as an in-depth discussion of the background, clinical presentation, diagnosis, and

Prim Care Clin Office Pract 50 (2023) xiii–xiv
https://doi.org/10.1016/j.pop.2023.01.004
0095-4543/23/© 2023 Published by Elsevier Inc.

management relevant to a primary care physician. We hope you find this update highly informative and enjoyable to read.

Andrew Lutzkanin III, MD, FAAFP
Department of Family and Community Medicine
Penn State College of Medicine
500 University Drive, H154
Hershey, PA 17033, USA

Kristen M. Lutzkanin, MD
Department of Pediatrics
Penn State College of Medicine
500 University Drive, H085
Hershey, PA 17033, USA

E-mail addresses:
alutzkanin@pennstatehealth.psu.edu (A. Lutzkanin)
klutzkanin@pennstatehealth.psu.edu (K.M. Lutzkanin)

Allergic Rhinitis

Eric J. Czech, MSBS, PA-C[a,b],*, Andrew Overholser, MSBS, PA-C[a,b],
Paul Schultz, MD[b]

KEYWORDS

- Allergic rhinitis • Histamine • Seasonal allergies • Allergen • Antihistamine
- Intranasal corticosteroids • Immunotherapy • Decongestant

KEY POINTS

- Allergic rhinitis is a common condition that can impact quality of life.
- Diagnosis of allergic rhinitis is largely based on history and physical examination.
- First-line treatment for allergic rhinitis is intranasal glucocorticosteroids.
- Allergen testing and desensitization immunotherapy (allergy shots) may be used for patients with chronic moderate-severe disease recalcitrant to first-line therapies.
- First-line therapies are available over the counter (eg, intranasal steroid sprays, antihistamines).

INTRODUCTION

Rhinitis is a common complaint in primary care, characterized by rhinorrhea, sneezing, congestion, cough, and nasal pruritus. Allergens are one of many rhinitis causes. Nonallergic rhinitis can occur from several mechanisms, including gustatory, vasomotor, irritants, medications, or various systemic diseases. Differentiating allergic versus nonallergic rhinitis is an essential skill for health care providers. Appropriate, accurate diagnosis and management can lead to increased quality of life and patient satisfaction.

EPIDEMIOLOGY

Approximately 10% to 20% of Americans are affected by allergic rhinitis, costing the US health care system $4.9 billion annually. Indirect costs can double this burden via lost work time, missed diagnosis, overprescribing, or secondary effects. This must be taken with a degree of skepticism, as while allergic rhinitis is a clinical diagnosis, further diagnostic options influence the data reported in several epidemiological studies.[1]

[a] Division of Physician Assistant Studies, Department of Family Medicine, The University of Toledo College of Medicine and Life Sciences, 3333 Glendale Avenue, Toledo, OH 43614, USA;
[b] Department of Family Medicine, The University of Toledo College of Medicine and Life Sciences, 3333 Glendale Avenue, Toledo, OH 43614, USA
* Corresponding author.
E-mail address: eric.czech@utoledo.edu

Prim Care Clin Office Pract 50 (2023) 159–178
https://doi.org/10.1016/j.pop.2023.01.003
0095-4543/23/© 2023 Elsevier Inc. All rights reserved.

PATHOPHYSIOLOGY

Upper airway allergic reactions occur primarily through a sequence of events in which allergens bind to specific receptors, prompting production of immunoglobulin E (IgE) and activating mast cells and basophils. Individuals must first become sensitized to an allergen before IgE is present. Histamine, prostaglandins, and leukotrienes play a role in the early phase response via activation of H1 receptors leading to pruritus, rhinorrhea, and sneezing. Prostaglandin and leukotrienes trigger release of vascular endothelial growth factors, contributing to increased vascular permeability and subsequent nasal congestion.[2] Late-phase responses include continued rhinorrhea and discharge of the nasal mucosa. The late phase response may continue and promote an influx of inflammatory cells, with an increased significance and duration.[2]

CLINICAL PRESENTATION

Allergic rhinitis is characterized by nasal congestion, nasal discharge, or rhinorrhea, with episodic, paroxysmal sneezing. Patients may also experience coughing, postnasal drip, nasal pruritus, conjunctival inflammation, and congestion of the upper airway, primarily in the nasal passages and maxillary and frontal sinuses.[3] Allergic rhinitis may be seasonal or perennial, mild, moderate, or severe. Allergic rhinitis is considered to be persistent when symptoms are present for greater than 4 times weekly over a period of longer than 4 weeks; conversely, allergic rhinitis with symptoms that occur less than 4 times weekly and last fewer than 4 weeks is considered intermittent.[4]

Variation in seasonal allergens causes differences between patients and the presentation of symptoms, with the need for management varying throughout the year. Investigations into pollen burden by region demonstrate changes in peak concentration and season duration and a variation of plant species between regions (**Table 1**). These factors influence the varied presentation of symptoms between geographic locations and individual patients.[5]

Patients with allergic rhinitis may also experience adverse effects on quality of life and cognitive performance. These primarily stem from altered breathing patterns leading to decreased sleep quality.[6] Sequelae of this phenomenon adversely affect cognitive performance and focus, resulting in general fatigue and daytime somnolence. Sequelae of allergic rhinitis have been linked to either the manifestation or exacerbation of attention deficit hyperactivity disorder in children and adolescents.[7]

Common associations with allergic rhinitis include atopic dermatitis, asthma, and food allergies. Thirty-eight percent of patients with allergic rhinitis are also afflicted with asthma.[8] Evidence suggests that symptoms of asthma can be exacerbated by allergic rhinitis itself, further complicating care. Comorbidities associated with allergic rhinitis include sinusitis, sleep pattern aberration, migraines, and gastroesophageal reflux.[9]

DIAGNOSTICS

Allergic rhinitis is a clinical diagnosis, rooted firmly in history and objective examination findings. Diagnosis is supported by classic symptoms of rhinorrhea, nasal congestion, sneezing paroxysms, nasal pruritus, cough, postnasal drip, and conjunctival inflammation. Presence of other atopic conditions supports the diagnosis. A thorough history should focus on symptom frequency and duration, specific symptoms and intensity, with previous therapies and their efficacy. Clinicians should assess at what time during the year allergic rhinitis symptoms are most prominent, if there are

Table 1
Average season start and length for common allergens in the United States

Allergens	Peak Season		Start Dates		Season Length
Oak	Spring	Northeast	Late April	Northeast	14–21 days
		Southeast	Early March	Southeast	35–45 days
		Midwest	Mid-April	Midwest	19–30 days
		Southwest	March–April	Southwest	27–45 days
		Northwest	Late April	Northwest	14–30 days
Birch (Betula)	Spring	Northeast	Late April	Northeast	29–35 days
		Southeast	Mid-February - early March	Southeast	35–40 days
		Midwest	Late March - late April	Midwest	29–36 days
		Southwest	–	Southwest	–
		Northwest	Late April	Northwest	27–34 days
Grass	Early summer	Northeast	Mid-April – mid-June	Northeast	37–91 days
		Southeast	Early March - mid April	Southeast	110–217 days
		Midwest	Mid-April - late May	Midwest	56–127 days
		Southwest	Mid-March - late May	Southwest	56–199 days
		Northwest	Mid-May – mid-June	Northwest	37–91 days
Ragweed	Late summer, autumn	Northeast	Late July - early August	Northeast	32–41 days
		Southeast	Late August – mid-September	Southeast	36–50 days
		Midwest	Late July – mid-August	Midwest	32–44 days
		Southwest	Mid-August – mid-September	Southwest	42–56 days
		Northwest	Late July - early August	Northwest	32–41 days
Mugwort	Late summer, autumn	Northeast	Early - late August	Northeast	39–46 days
		Southeast	Late August - late September	Southeast	29–46 days
		Midwest	Mid July - late August	Midwest	29–46 days
		Southwest	Late August - late September	Southwest	24–46 days
		Northwest	Mid July - early September	Northwest	8–43 days

Adapted from Zhang Y, Bielory L, Cai T, Mi Z, Georgopoulos P. Predicting onset and duration of airborne allergenic pollen season in the United States. Atmos Environ (1994). 2015;103:297–306.

any known exacerbating triggers such as occupational exposures or pet dander, and if previously trialed treatments were effective.[10]

Physical examination of the patient with allergic rhinitis should include an assessment of the eyes, ears, nose, and throat. Pale, boggy, edematous nasal mucosa are common in allergic rhinitis, with a 67% sensitivity and 37% specificity. Nasal turbinate hypertrophy carries a 90% sensitivity but only a 2.3% specificity.[11] Examination of the eyes may reveal lacrimation and inflamed conjunctiva, while the oropharynx may demonstrate postnasal drip or a cobblestone appearance.[10]

Patients may demonstrate various physical findings of allergic rhinitis, including morning Dennie-Morgan lines (creases or folds inferior to the lower eyelids), infraorbital edema and darkening known as allergic shiners, or nasal polyps.[10] Nasal polyps carry a 95% specificity but only a 12% sensitivity.[11]

Qualifying allergic rhinitis into severity categories influences therapeutic intensity. Classic categories are mild or moderate-severe. Mild allergic rhinitis is associated with absence of alteration in daily activities, sleep, performance in work or school-type environments, and a lack of overall troubling symptoms. The diagnosis of moderate-severe allergic rhinitis can be established with aberrations in normal sleep patterns, daily routines or activities, adverse effects on cognitive performance, or overall troublesome symptoms.[10] Symptoms and severity of allergic rhinitis can progress over time. Patients may move between mild or moderate-severe allergic rhinitis throughout the disease process.

Additional laboratory testing is available to confirm and specify responsible allergens. To identify allergen triggers, serum IgE levels to environmental allergens can be assessed in primary care. Skin prick testing can be done in an allergist's office. The more specific diagnosis of local allergic rhinitis can be confirmed with the presence of IgE in nasal secretions, although this is rarely done.[12]

MANAGEMENT/THERAPEUTICS

Allergic rhinitis usually requires pharmacological therapy to control symptoms. Often, patients can only minimally change or control their environment. Many pharmacological therapies for allergic rhinitis are available over the counter, and patients tend to try their own therapies (**Table 2**). This can cause overuse of first-generation antihistamines and the underuse of intranasal corticosteroids. Some concerns leading to underutilization of intranasal corticosteroids include safety and efficacy, confusing intranasal corticosteroids with decongestants, cost, undesirable feelings of intranasal use, and inability to feel a result quickly.[13]

Allergen Avoidance

The best method to control allergic rhinitis is prevention by avoiding allergens. If practical, the patient and provider should develop avoidance strategies to minimize or eliminate exposure to causative agents. Patients frequently have multiple environmental allergens, making meaningful avoidance difficult to achieve. A summary of avoidance strategies is presented in **Fig. 1**.[14]

Allergen Immunotherapy

Once specific triggering allergens are determined, under the treatment of an allergist, a patient can have desensitizing immunotherapy to reduce symptoms and the need for chronic medication. Immunotherapy is usually deployed with either subcutaneous immunotherapy (SCIT) or sublingual immunotherapy (SLIT). Only a few allergens have been standardized with dosing and extracts, as discussed in **Table 2**.[1] Using

Table 2
Summary of medical therapy for allergic rhinitis

Class and Receptors Effected	Generic Name	Brand Name	Therapy Changing Adverse/Side Effects	Prescription Required?	Generic Available?	Pediatric Dosing	Adult Dosing	Other Mechanisms of Action?	Use in Pregnancy?	Other
First Generation Intra-Nasal Corticosteroids (Bioavailability 10%–50%)	Beclomethasone dipropionate nasal	Beconase AQ (42 μg/spray)	Potential for hypercortisicm	Yes	No	Age 6–11 y: Start 1 spray each nostril twice daily. May increase to 1 to 2 sprays each nostril twice daily Age >12 y: 1 to 2 sprays each nostril twice daily	1–2 sprays each nostril twice daily		Yes	
		Qnasl Childrens (40 μg/spray)	Potential for hypercortisicm	Yes	No	4–11 y: 1 spray each nostril daily			Yes	
		Qnasl (80 μg/spray)	Potential for hypercortisicm	Yes	No	>12 y: 2 sprays each nostril daily	2 sprays each nostril daily		Yes	
	Budesonide nasal	Rhinocort Allergy (32 μg/spray)	Potential for hypercortisicm	No	Yes	Age 6–11 y: Start 1 spray each nostril once daily. May increase to 1 to 2 sprays each nostril once daily Age >12 y: 1 to 2 sprays each nostril once daily	1–2 sprays each nostril daily		Yes, preferred agent	
	Flunisolide nasal	Nasarel (25 μg/spray)	Potential for hypercortisicm	Yes	Yes	Age 6–14 y: 2 sprays each nostril twice daily Age >15 y: 2 sprays each nostril two–three times daily	2 sprays each nostril 2–3 times daily		Yes	
	Triamcinolone nasal	Nasacort Allergy 24 h (55 μg/spray)	Potential for hypercortisicm	No	Yes	Age 2–5 y: 1 spray each nostril once daily Age 6–11 y: Start 1 spray each nostril once daily. May increase to 1 to 2 sprays each nostril once daily Age >12 y: 1–2 sprays each nostril once daily	2 sprays each nostril once daily		Yes	

(continued on next page)

Table 2
(continued)

Class and Receptors Effected	Generic Name	Brand Name	Therapy Changing Adverse/Side Effects	Prescription Required?	Generic Available?	Pediatric Dosing	Adult Dosing	Other Mechanisms of Action?	Use in Pregnancy?	Other
Second-generation intranasal corticosteroids (Bioavailability <1%)	Ciclesonide nasal	Omnaris (50 µg/spray)	Lower theoretical potential for hypercortisicm as compared to first generation	Yes	No	Age 2–11 y: 1 to 2 sprays each nostril once daily; Age >12 y: 2 sprays each nostril once daily	2 sprays each nostril daily		Yes	
		Zetonna (37 µg/spray)	Lower theoretical potential for hypercortisicm as compared to first generation	Yes	No	Age >12 y: 1 spray each nostril once daily	1 spray each nostril daily		Yes	
	Fluticasone propionate nasal	Xhance (93 µg/spray)	Lower theoretical potential for hypercortisicm as compared to first generation	Yes	No		1–2 sprays each nostril twice daily		Yes	
		Flonase (50 µg/spray)	Lower theoretical potential for hypercortisicm as compared to first generation	No	Yes	Age 4–11 y: 1 spray each nostril once daily; Age >12 y: 2 sprays each nostril once daily	1–2 sprays each nostril daily		Yes	
	Fluticasone furoate nasal	Flonase Sensimist (27.5 µg/spray)	Lower theoretical potential for hypercortisicm as compared to first generation	No	No	Age 2–11 y: 1 spray each nostril once daily; Age >12 y: 1–2 sprays each nostril once daily	2 sprays each nostril daily		Yes	Taking with a CYP3A4 inhibitor will increase fluticasone blood levels
	Momentasone nasal	Nasonex *50 µg/spray	Lower theoretical potential for hypercortisicm as compared to first generation	No	Yes	Age 2–11 y: 1 spray each nostril once daily; Age >12 y: 1–2 sprays each nostril once daily	2 sprays each nostril daily		Yes	

	Generic	Brand	Sedation			Pediatric dosing	Adult dosing		Notes
second-generation antihistimines (histimine-1 peripheral receptor antagonist)	Loratadine	Claratin	Low potential for sedation	No	Yes	Age 2–5 y: 5 mg by mouth daily Age >6 y: 10 mg by mouth daily	10 mg once daily	Yes	
	Desloratadine	Clarinex	Low potential for sedation	Yes	No	Age 6–11 mo: 1 mg by mouth daily Age 1–5 y: 1.25 mg by mouth daily Age 6–11 y: 2.5 mg by mouth daily Age >12 y: 5 mg by mouth daily	5mg once daily	Yes	
	Cetirizine	Zytec	Higher risk of sedation as compared to other second gen antihistamines (10% of patients)	No	Yes	Age 6–11 mo: 2.5 mg by mouth daily Age 12–23 mo: 2.5 mg by mouth daily or twice daily Age 2–5 y: 5 mg by mouth daily. Start 2.5 mg by mouth daily.	10 mg once daily Age > 65 y: 5 mg by mouth daily	Yes	
	Levocetirizine	Xyzal	Low potential for sedation	Yes	No	Age >6 y: 5–10 mg by mouth daily Age 6–11 y: 2.5 mg by mouth nightly Age >12 y: 2.5–5 mg by mouth nightly	2.5–5 mg once daily at bedtime	Yes	
		Children's Xyzal (2.5 mg/5 mL solution)	Low potential for sedation	Yes	No	Age 2–5 y: 2.5 mL by mouth nightly Age 6–11 y: 5 mL by mouth nightly Age 12–18 y: 5–10 mL by mouth nightly Age >65 y: 5 mL by mouth nightly		Yes	
Third-generation antihistimines (histimine-1 peripheral receptor antagonist)	Fexofenadine	Allegra		No	Yes	Age 2–11 y: 30 mg by mouth daily Age >12 y: 180 mg by mouth daily	180 mg once daily	Yes	Taking with juice (fruit juice) will lower blood levels

(continued on next page)

Table 2
(continued)

Class and Receptors Effected	Generic Name	Brand Name	Prescription Required?	Generic Available?	Therapy Changing Adverse/Side Effects	Pediatric Dosing	Adult Dosing	Other Mechanisms of Action?	Use in Pregnancy?	Other
Intranasal antihistimines (histimine-1 peripheral/central nervous system [CNS] receptor antagonst)	Olopatadine nasal	Patanase (660 μg/spray) 0.6%	Yes	No		Age 6–11 y: 1 spray each nostril twice daily; Age >12 y: 1–2 sprays each nostril twice daily	2 sprays each nostri twice daily	Antihistimine, Mast cell stabilizer, and anti-inflammatory effects	Yes	
	Azelastine nasal	Astepro (205.5 μg/spray) 0.15%	No	No		Age 6–11 y: 1 spray each nostril twice daily; Age >12 y: 1–2 sprays each nostril twice daily	1–2 sprays each nostril daily	Antihistimine and anti-inflammatory effects	Yes	
Intranasal mast cell stabilizer	Cromolyn sodium	Nasalcrom 5.2 mg/spray	No	No		Age 2 years and older: 1 sprays each nostril three-four times daily. Max 1 spray each nostril six times daily	1 sprays each nostril three-four times daily. Max 1 spray each nostril six times daily		Yes	Limited efficacy. May be tried. Very safe to use
Antileukotriene agents (leukotriene receptor antagonist)	Montelukast	Singulair	Yes	Yes	Serious neuropsychiatric effects seen. Alternative therapies now recommended based on benefit/risk ratio	Age 6–23 mo: 4 mg by mouthevery day; Age 2–5 y: 4 mg by mouth every day; Age 6–14 y: 5 mg by mouth every day; Age >15 y: 10 mg by mouth everyday	10 mg by mouth daily		Probably not	Can use if other agents do not work.
Systemic corticosteroids (ie, prednisone)	Prednisone	Deltasone	Yes	Yes	Higher potential for hypercortisicm as compared to topical preparations	0.05–2 mg/kg/day by mouth divided once-four times daily	5–60 mg by mouth daily		Yes	Not recommended for mild/moderate cases. Use for shortest duration
	Methylprednisolone	Medrol	Yes	Yes	Higher potential for hypercortisicm as compared to topical preparations	0.5–1.7 mg/kg/day by mouth divided every 6–12h	4–48 mg/day by mouth divided once-four times daily		Yes	Not recommended for mild/moderate cases. Use for shortest duration

Intranasal anticholinergics (muscarinic receptor antagonist)	Ipratropium bromide	Atrovent Nasal (21g/spray) 0.06%	Anticholinergic	Yes	Yes	Age 5 years and older: 2 sprays each nostril four times daily	2 sprays each nostril four times daily		Yes	May help with rhinorrhea if uncontrolled on other agents (topical glucocorticoids)
First-generation antihistamines (histimine-1 peripheral/CNS receptor antagonist, muscarinic receptor antagonist)	Diphenhydramine	Benadryl	Sedation, anticholinergic	No	Yes	Age 2-5 y: 6.25 mg by mouth every 4-6 h. Max 37.5 mg daily Age 6-11 y: 12.5-25 mg by mouth every 4-6 h. Max 150 mg daily. Age >12 y: 25-50 mg every 2-6 h. Max 300 mg daily.	25-50 mg by mouth every 2-6 h. Max 300 mg daily Limit use >65 y old patients	Intracellar sodium channel blocker (Can produce local anesthesia)	Yes	Age 2-11 y: For severe symptoms: 1-2 mg/kg/dose every 6 h as needed. Max 50 mg/dose and 300 mg daily
	Dimenhydrinate (diphenhydramine/ 8-chlorotheophylline)	Dramamine	Sedation, anticholinergic	No	Yes	Age 2-5 y: 12.5-25 mg by mouth every 6-8 h. Max 75 mg daily. Age 6-11 y: 25-50 mg by mouth every 6-8 h. Max 150 mg daily. Age >12 y: 50-100 mg every 4-6 h. Max 600 mg daily.	50-100 mg by mouth every 4-6 h. Max 600 mg daily. Limit use >65 y old patients	Intracellar sodium channel blocker (Can produce local anesthesia)	Yes	8-chlorotheophylline is a xanthine derivative, such as caffeine. It is combined with diphenhydramine in an attempt to counteract the sedative effects
	Doxylamine	Vick's ZzzQuil Ultra Unisom Sleep Tabs	Sedation, anticholinergic	No	Yes	Age >12 y: 12.5 mg by mouth every 4-6 h. Max 75 mg daily	12.5 mg by mouth every 4-6 h. Max 75 mg daily Limit use >65 y old patients		Yes	
	Chlorpheniramine	Aller-Chlor	Sedation, anticholinergic	No	Yes	Age 6-11 y: 2 mg by mouth every 6-8 h. Max 12 mg daily. Age >12 y: 4 mg every 4-6 h. Max 24 mg daily.	4mg by mouth every 4-6 h. Max 24 mg daily Limit use >65 y old patients		Yes	

(continued on next page)

Table 2
(continued)

Class and Receptors Effected	Generic Name	Brand Name	Therapy Changing Adverse/Side Effects	Prescription Required?	Generic Available?	Pediatric Dosing	Adult Dosing	Other Mechanisms of Action?	Use in Pregnancy?	Other
	Brompheniramine	Children's Dimetapp (Brompheniramine/Phenylephrine 2 mg-5 mg/10 mL)	Sedation, anticholinergic	No	No	Age 6-11 y: 10 mL by mouth every 4 h. Max 60 mL daily. Age >12 y: 10 mL every 4 h. Max 120 mL daily.			No	Only available in combination with phenylephrine.
	Promethazine	Phenergan	Sedation, anticholinergic, extrapyramidal symptoms, orthostatic hypotension	Yes	Yes	Age 2 years and older: 0.1 mg/kg/dose by mouth every 6 h. Max 12.5 mg/dose during day, 25 mg/dose at night, 100 mg daily.	6.25-25 mg by mouth three-four times daily. Max 100 mg daily. Limit use >65 y old patients	Dopamine-2 Receptor Antagonist, Alpha-1 Adrenergic Receptor Antagonist	Probably not. Risk of fetal respiratory depression	
	Hydroxyzine	Atarax	Sedation, less anticholinergic	Yes	Yes	Age <6 y: 2 mg/kg/day by mouth divided every 6-8 h Age 6-12 y: 2 mg/kg/day by mouth divided every 6-8 h Age >12 y: 25 mg by mouth every 6-8 h.	25 mg by mouth every 6-8 h. Limit use >65 y old patients	Weak antagonist at Serotonin 5-HT2a, Dopamine D2, and alpha-1 adrenergic receptors.	Proabably	Less anti-cholinergic action than diphenhydramine
	Carbinoxamine	Karbinal ER	Sedation, anticholinergic	Yes	Yes	Age 2-3 y: 0.2-0.4 mg/kg/day by mouth divided every 12 h Age 4-5 y: 0.2-0.4 mg/kg/day by mouth divided every 12 h Age 6-11 y: 0.2-0.4 mg/kg/day by mouth divided every 12 h Age >12 y: 6-16 mg by mouth every 12 h.	6-16 mg by mouth every 12 h. Limit use >65 y old patients		Yes	

Drug	Brand	Side effects		Pediatric dose	Adult dose	Mechanism		Comments
Clemastine		Sedation, anticholinergic	No	Age 6–11 y: 0.5–1 mg by mouth twice-three times daily. Max 3 mg daily. Age >12 y: 1–2 mg by mouth twice-three times daily. Max 6 mg daily.	1–2 mg by mouth twice daily. Max 6 mg daily Limit use >65 y old patients		Yes	
Cyproheptadine	Periactin	Sedation, anticholinergic	Yes	Age 6–11 y: 2 mg by mouth every 8–12h. Max 3 mg daily. Age 7–14 y: 4 mg by mouth every 8–12h Max 6 mg daily.	4mg by mouth three times daily. Max 0.5 mg/kg/day Limit use >65 y old patients	Serotonin 5-HT1 antagonist, 5-HT2 antagonist, possible antiandrogenic.	Yes	
Triprolidine	Histex	Sedation, anticholinergic	No	Age 6–11 y: 1.25 mg by mouth every 4–6 h. Max 5 mg daily Age >12 y: 2.5 mg by mouth every 4–6 h. Max 10 mg daily			No	
Decongestants, oral (alpha-1 adrenergic agonists) Phenylephrine	Sudafed-PE	Hypertension, insomnia, irritability, headache, rebound nasal congestion	No	Age >12 y: 10 mg by mouth every 4–6 h. Max 60 mg daily	10 mg by mouth every 4–6 h. Max 60 mg daily		No	Not recommended monotherapy. Do not use longer than 3 days
Pseudoephedrine	Sudafed	Hypertension, insomnia, irritability, headache, rebound nasal congestion	No	Age 2–3 y: 15 mg by mouth every 4–6 hr. Max 60 mg daily Age 4–5 y: 15 mg by mouth every 4–6 hr. Max 60 mg daily Age 6–11 y: 30 mg by mouth every 4–6 hr. Max 120 mg daily Age >12 y: 60 mg by mouth every 4–6 h. Max 240 mg daily	60 mg by mouth every 4–6 h. Max 240 mg daily		No	Not recommended monotherapy. Do not use longer than 3 days

(continued on next page)

Table 2
(continued)

Class and Receptors Effected	Generic Name	Brand Name	Therapy Changing Adverse/Side Effects	Prescription Required?	Generic Available?	Pediatric Dosing	Adult Dosing	Other Mechanisms of Action?	Use in Pregnancy?	Other
Intranasal decongestants (alpha-1 Adrenergic agonists)	Oxymetazoline	Afrin Nasal Spray 0.05%	Hypertension, insomnia, irritability, headache, rebound nasal congestion	No	Yes	Age >6 y: 2–3 sprays in each nostril q10–12 h	2–3 sprays in each nostril q10–12 h		Yes	Not recommended monotherapy. Do not use longer than 3 days
	Phenylephrine	Neo-synephrine Nasal Spray 1%	Hypertension, insomnia, irritability, headache, rebound nasal congestion	No	Yes		2–3 sprays in each nostril every 4 h		Proabably not	Not recommended monotherapy. Do not use longer than 3 days

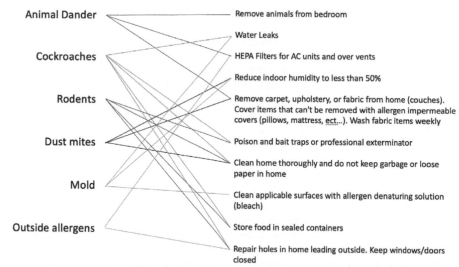

Fig. 1. Common indoor allergens and allergen avoidance strategies. (*Adapted from* Platts-Mills TA. Allergen avoidance in the treatment of asthma and allergic rhinitis. Uptodate.com, 2021, Available at: https://www.uptodate.com/contents/allergen-avoidance-in-the-treatment-of-asthma-and-allergic-rhinitis?search=Allergen%20avoidance%20in%20the%20treatment%20of%20asthma%20and%20allergic%20rhinitis&source=search_result&selectedTitle=1~150&usage_type=default&display_rank=1, Accessed September 27, 2022.)

SLIT may provide a less invasive route of administration and increase patient compliance, but current data suggest that SCIT may be more efficacious than SLIT. Head-to-head trials are lacking, however, and further research is needed.[15]

Nasal Saline

Irrigation with sterile saline can aid in cleansing the nasal cavity of allergens. This is generally recommended for mild allergic rhinitis. Administration of nasal saline can be through over-the-counter bottles, Nettie Potts, syringes, or electronic devices. It is important to use sterile saline and not tap water or another nonsterile solution to prevent entry of foreign microbes and material into the nasal cavity. Isotonic nasal saline irrigation is an effective adjunctive or monotherapy for mild allergic rhinitis when compared with intranasal corticosteroids.[16]

Glucocorticoid Nasal Sprays

Glucocorticoid nasal sprays are the most effective monotherapy agent and are the mainstay of treatment for allergic rhinitis, with adverse effects at recommended doses.[17,18]

Agent Selection

Specific agents are listed in **Table 2**. Studies fail to demonstrate any significant differences in efficacy of one agent over another. Therefore, when prescribing these medications, care should be taken regarding comorbidities and bioavailability of the corticosteroid. First-generation corticosteroids have significantly higher systemic bioavailability than second-generation; however, the risk of systemic adverse effects for first-generation or second-generation formulations is low. A potential worrisome side effect would be hypercorticism, which can lead to hypothalamic pituitary adrenal axis suppression. Fortunately, multiple studies with first- and second-generation corticosteroids have shown hypothalamic pituitary adrenal axis suppression does not occur with long-term use.[19,20] Other major concerns related to intranasal use of glucocorticosteroids include slow growth in children, promotion of osteopenia, osteoporosis, glaucoma, and cataracts. A 2020 practice guideline review on allergic rhinitis and multiple studies failed to show any significant adverse effects of long-term intranasal corticosteroid use in children and adults.[5,21–24] Class-wide adverse effects including taste change, burning, dryness, and epistaxis are less concerning for long-term harm but may lead to patient intolerance and treatment cessation. Perforation of the nasal septum has been a reported complication, but incidence is low.[20] Epistaxis with intranasal corticosteroid use is seen in 5% to 10% of patients, most likely the result of mucosal irritation and minor trauma. Trace blood in mucosal secretions should be expected. Stopping treatment for a couple of days can mitigate these symptoms. In patients with persistent and/or severe epistaxis, workup for other causes should ensue, and stopping therapy may be warranted with transition to other alternatives.[25]

Most of the onset of action is within a few hours; maximal effect occurs within 2 days to 3 weeks.[26] Patients may believe the medication is not working, because effects are not immediate. Proper education on onset of action and use of these medications is important for compliance.[27] It is recommended to start therapy at the highest dose based on age, tapering down to the lowest effective dose after symptom control.

Administration of Intranasal Corticosteroids

Proper administration of intranasal corticosteroids depends on patients' ability to self-administer. The head should be pointed downward while spraying, preventing excess corticosteroids from draining down the throat; patients should spray away from the nasal septum. If the patient has significant congestion preventing effective administration and coating of the mucosa, temporary use of a decongestant spray before intranasal corticosteroid administration can increase corticosteroid penetrance.[28,29]

Antihistamines

When comparing the efficacy of oral antihistamines against intranasal corticosteroids, intranasal corticosteroids are significantly more efficacious than antihistamines, reducing total nasal symptom score by 25% more than the control, whereas antihistamines have. decreased total nasal symptoms by up to 10%.[30,31] A 2020 practice parameter update recommends starting therapy for intermittent allergic rhinitis with either an intranasal corticosteroid or oral antihistamine. Patients with persistent symptomatically mild allergic rhinitis should start with an intranasal corticosteroid and use an oral antihistamine if symptoms are not controlled. Adding oral antihistamines to intranasal glucocorticoids provides no additional benefit.[5]

First-Generation Antihistamines

First-generation antihistamines are widely available; however, potential adverse effects limit their use. These drugs can cross the blood-brain barrier and antagonize central nervous system histamine-1 receptors, causing sedative side effects.[5] In addition, they have a varying affinity for antagonizing peripheral and central muscarinic receptors, leading to significant anticholinergic side effects.[5] This is particularly important when using antihistamines in older patients who may have a higher risk of falls or dizziness associated with central antagonism of histamine.[5] Furthermore, anticholinergic side effects in older patients can include urinary retention, constipation, delirium, tachycardia, and increased intraocular pressure.[32] A 2015 study also correlated the risk of chronic anticholinergic use with dementia.[33] First-generation antihistamines are not recommended for allergic rhinitis in favor of second and third-generation nonsedating antihistamines.[5]

Second- and Third-Generation Antihistamines

Second-generation and third-generation antihistamines are more lipophobic than first-generation antihistamines, decreasing their adverse effects. Although second-generation antihistamines are less sedating, cetirizine can be sedating in up to 10% of patients.[34] Also, there can be varying levels of anticholinergic adverse effects in some patients, although they tend to be less than first-generation antihistamines.[35] Although not superior to intranasal glucocorticoids, second- and third-generation antihistamines are recommended for use in allergic rhinitis.[5] There is no evidence to suggest that tolerance develops with antihistamines, allowing for chronic use.[36]

Intranasal Antihistamines

Intranasal antihistamines have significant clinical benefits in allergic rhinitis along with anti-inflammatory effects.[37] Olopatadine is shown to have antihistamine, mast cell stabilizing, and anti-inflammatory properties.[38] Benefits of intranasal antihistamines may include an onset of action within 15 minutes, although maximum efficacy occurs in 2 to 3 days.[39] When comparing the efficacy of intranasal antihistamines and intranasal corticosteroids, many studies favor corticosteroids.[40] Some studies suggest intranasal antihistamines have comparable efficacy to intranasal corticosteroids.[41,42] There is no statistical benefit of choosing an intranasal antihistamine over an oral antihistamine other than choosing targeted versus systemic therapy.[43]

Intranasal Mast Cell Stabilizer

Cromolyn sodium is the only intranasal mast cell stabilizer available in the United States and reduces mast cell histamine release. Use is limited because of low efficacy and is relegated to an adjunctive role in some cases of mild allergic rhinitis.[44]

Antileukotriene agents

Leukotriene receptor antagonists like montelukast are moderately effective in treating allergic rhinitis and are similar in efficacy to oral antihistamines.[45,46] Other studies suggest that leukotriene receptor antagonists are moderately less effective than oral antihistamines,[47,48] and are far less efficacious than intranasal corticosteroids.[48,49] Previously, montelukast was widely used in combination with oral antihistamines to provide additional benefit for allergic rhinitis. This is not favorable because of increased neuropsychiatric adverse effects.[50,51] The US Food and Drug Administration (FDA) released a black box warning for montelukast because of increases in these adverse effects in pediatric, adolescent, and adult patients. Adverse effects can include vivid dreams, depression with suicidal thoughts, insomnia, disorientation, aggression, hallucinations, obsessive-compulsive symptoms, tics, and memory impairment.[52] When considering this medication for allergic rhinitis, shared decision making regarding the risks and benefits of treatment is advised. Antileukotriene agents can benefit patients with concurrent asthma that is not well controlled. Leukotriene receptor antagonists are not recommended for initial treatment of allergic rhinitis. They are best reserved as adjunctive treatment in combination therapy based on careful risk-benefit analysis.[52]

Systemic Corticosteroids

Systemic corticosteroids may be used for a short treatment course of severe and/or intractable allergic rhinitis over 5 to 7 days. This allows time for other agents to take effect. The recommendation is to use the lowest dose for the shortest amount of time because of potential adverse effects.[53]

Oral and Intranasal Decongestants

Oral decongestants such as phenylephrine and pseudoephedrine act as peripheral alpha-adrenergic agonists, relieving nasal congestion and rhinorrhea through vaso-constriction.[54] Unfortunately, oral phenylephrine is ineffective at treating nasal congestion at doses up to 40 mg when compared with placebo.[54] Class adverse effects include elevated blood pressure, insomnia, appetite suppression, irritability, and palpitations. Cautious consideration of these agents in those with cardiac comorbidities, thyroid disease, glaucoma, benign prostatic hyperplasia, psychiatric conditions, and cerebrovascular disease is advised.[54]

Many topical nasal decongestants are available with vasoconstrictive activity. They are effective for nasal congestion. Use is limited for symptom relief to 3 days because of the risk of rhinitis medicamentosa. Proper use of topical nasal decongestants combined with topical corticosteroids can more effectively treat the symptoms of rhinitis and nasal congestion without the risk of rhinitis medicamentosa.[53]

Intranasal Anticholinergics

Ipratropium bromide is the only available anticholinergic nasal spray and can be effective in decreasing rhinorrhea. It is significantly less efficacious than intranasal corticosteroids for sneezing, pruritus, and nasal congestion.[44] It is not recommended as a first-line treatment for allergic rhinitis because of limited efficacy compared with other agents. This agent should only be used in those with allergic rhinitis where rhinorrhea is not controlled with first-line agents.[44]

SUMMARY

Allergic rhinitis is common in primary care, affecting up to 20% of Americans. It can have a variable presentation with IgE-mediated symptoms including runny nose, congestion, sneezing, mucosal pruritus, postnasal drip, and conjunctival inflammation. Diagnosis is typically made on history and physical examination. At this initial stage, laboratory and/or imaging studies are not generally needed. Ruling out other etiologies with similar presentations is often challenging. Reassessment of alternative diagnoses is important when treatments are ineffective. When allergic rhinitis is mild, properly performed nasal saline rinses provide significant relief. In both mild and moderate-severe allergic rhinitis, first-line treatment with intranasal glucocorticoid sprays can provide symptom improvement. Educating patients in proper technique to administer nasal spray can optimize drug efficacy. An alternative treatment shown to provide benefit either as monotherapy or in combination with steroid nasal spray is a second- or third-generation antihistamine. First-generation antihistamines are not first-line options because of potential side effects of sedation and urinary retention. Leukotriene receptor antagonists can reduce the inflammatory response in nasal and respiratory mucosa. These continue to be an option for adjunctive therapy in patients with associated asthma. When nasal steroid sprays and/or second-generation antihistamines are insufficient, and symptoms are at a level to create secondary effects (eg, fatigue, cognitive impairment, sleep disruption), allergen testing can be performed. Once triggering allergens are identified, desensitizing immunotherapy (allergy shots) can reduce symptom burden. At initiation of treatment, use of temporary symptom relief measures such as intranasal or systemic decongestants can provide benefit while waiting for intranasal glucocorticoids to become effective. In more severe presentations, a short,

5- to 7-day course of oral corticosteroids can be considered while waiting for first-line treatments to become therapeutic. A shared decision-making approach incorporating a risk-benefit discussion and patient education is advisable.

CLINICS CARE POINTS

- Allergic rhinitis is an IgE-mediated immune response to environmental allergens.
- Diagnosis is achieved through history and physical examination; testing is not usually needed.
- Other conditions can overlap with allergic rhinitis. If first-line therapies are not effective, reconsider the differential diagnoses.
- For known allergens, avoidance measures can provide a cost-effective, low-risk benefit.
- Recommend nasal saline rinses, as these reduce symptoms.
- Intranasal corticosteroid sprays are the most efficacious first-line therapy.
- Educate patients to spray up toward the sinuses, away from the nasal septum, while performing a coordinated subtle sniff to ensure medication will be delivered to the nasal mucosa.
- Second- or third-generation antihistamines are also effective either in monotherapy or in combination with nasal steroid sprays.
- Although many options are available over the counter, patients may fail to optimize these medications. Patient education on treatment options, mechanisms of action, and treatment goals is essential.
- First-generation antihistamines can provide symptom relief but are best avoided, particularly in the geriatric population, because of increased adverse effect potential.
- Allergen testing and desensitizing immunotherapy are best reserved for those recalcitrant to first-line therapy options and/or those who have moderate-severe symptoms impacting quality of life.

DISCLOSURE

The authors have nothing to disclose.

REFERENCES

1. Mims JW. Epidemiology of allergic rhinitis. Int Forum Allergy Rhinol 2014;4(S2): S18–20.
2. Eifan AO, Durham SR. Pathogenesis of rhinitis. Clin Exp Allergy 2016;46(9): 1139–51.
3. Ng MLS, Warlow RS, Chrishanthan N, et al. Preliminary criteria for the definition of allergic rhinitis: a systematic evaluation of clinical parameters in a disease cohort (I). Clin Exp Allergy 2000;30(9):1314–31.
4. Bousquet J, Khaltaev N, Cruz AA, et al. Allergic rhinitis and its impact on asthma (ARIA) 2008*. Allergy 2008;63(s86):8–160.
5. Zhang Y, Bielorya L, Caia T, et al. Predicting onset and duration of airborne allergenic pollen season in the United States. Atmos Environ 1994;103:297–306.
6. Koinis-Mitchell D, Craig T, Esteban CA, et al. Sleep and allergic disease: a summary of the literature and future directions for research. J Allergy Clin Immunol 2012;130(6):1275–81.

7. Brawley A, Silverman B, Kearney S, et al. Allergic rhinitis in children with attention-deficit/hyperactivity disorder. Ann Allergy Asthma Immunol 2004;92(6):663–7.

8. Acevedo-Prado A, Seoane-Pillado T, López-Silvarrey-Varela A, et al. Association of rhinitis with asthma prevalence and severity. Sci Rep 2022;12(1). https://doi.org/10.1038/s41598-022-10448-w.

9. Hadley JA, Derebery MJ, Marple BF. Comorbidities and allergic rhinitis: Not just a runny nose. J Fam Pract 2012;61(2):S11–5.

10. Ryan D. How to identify and manage seasonal allergic rhinitis. J Community Nurs 2016;30(2):54–9.

11. Eren E, Aktaş A, Arslanoğlu S, et al. Diagnosis of allergic rhinitis: inter-rater reliability and predictive value of nasal endoscopic examination: a prospective observational study. Clin Otolaryngol 2013;38(6):481–6.

12. Krzych-Fałta E, Wojas O, Samoliński BK, et al. Gold standard diagnostic algorithm for the differential diagnosis of local allergic rhinitis. Postepy Dermatol Alergol 2022;39(1):20–5.

13. Bridgeman MB. Overcoming barriers to intranasal corticosteroid use in patients with uncontrolled allergic rhinitis. Integr Pharm Res Pract 2017;6:109–19.

14. Platts-Mills TA. Allergen avoidance in the treatment of asthma and allergic rhinitis. Uptodate.com 2021. Available at: https://www.uptodate.com/contents/allergen-avoidance-in-the-treatment-of-asthma-and-allergic-rhinitis?search=Allergen%20avoidance%20in%20the%20treatment%20of%20asthma%20and%20allergic%20rhinitis&source=search_result&selectedTitle=1~150&usage_type=default&display_rank=1. Accessed September 27, 2022.

15. Tabatabaian F, Casale TB. Selection of patients for sublingual immunotherapy (SLIT) versus subcutaneous immunotherapy (SCIT). Allergy Asthma Proc 2015;36(2):100–4.

16. Nguyen SA, Psaltis AJ, Schlosser RJ. Isotonic saline nasal irrigation is an effective adjunctive therapy to intranasal corticosteroid spray in allergic rhinitis. Am J Rhinol Allergy 2014;28(4):308–11.

17. Wallace DV, Dykewicz MS, Oppenheimer J, et al. Pharmacologic treatment of seasonal allergic rhinitis: synopsis of guidance from the 2017 joint task force on practice parameters. Ann Intern Med 2017;167(12):876–81.

18. Small P, Keith PK, Kim H. Allergic rhinitis. Allergy Asthma Clin Immunol 2018;14(2):51.

19. Fowler J, Rotenberg BW, Sowerby LJ. The subtle nuances of intranasal corticosteroids. J Otolaryngol Head Neck Surg 2021;50(1):18.

20. Dykewicz MS, Wallace DV, Amrol DJ, et al. Rhinitis 2020: a practice parameter update. J Allergy Clin Immunol 2020;146(4):721–67.

21. Juniper EF, Ståhl E, Doty RL, et al. Clinical outcomes and adverse effect monitoring in allergic rhinitis. J Allergy Clin Immunol 2005;115(3 Suppl 1):S390–413.

22. Schenkel EJ, Skoner DP, Bronsky EA, et al. Absence of growth retardation in children with perennial allergic rhinitis after one year of treatment with mometasone furoate aqueous nasal spray. Pediatrics 2000;105(2):E22.

23. Galant SP, Melamed IR, Nayak AS, et al. Lack of effect of fluticasone propionate aqueous nasal spray on the hypothalamic-pituitary-adrenal axis in 2- and 3-year-old patients. Pediatrics 2003;112:96–100.

24. Benninger MS, Ahmad N, Marple BF. The safety of intranasal steroids. J Otolaryngol Head Neck Surg 2003;129(6):739–50.

25. Wu EL, Harris WC, Babcock CM, et al. Epistaxis risk associated with intranasal corticosteroid sprays: a systematic review and meta-analysis. J Otolaryngol Head Neck Surg 2019;161(1):18–27.

26. Patel D, Garadi R, Brubaker M, et al. Onset and duration of action of nasal sprays in seasonal allergic rhinitis patients: olopatadine hydrochloride versus mometasone furoate monohydrate. Allergy Asthma Proc 2007;28(5):592–9.
27. Loh CY, Chao SS, Chan YH, et al. A clinical survey on compliance in the treatment of rhinitis using nasal steroids. Allergy 2004;59(11):1168–72.
28. Khattiyawittayakun L, Seresirikachorn K, Chitsuthipakorn W, et al. Effects of decongestant addition to intranasal corticosteroid for chronic rhinitis: a systematic review and meta-analysis. Int Forum Allergy Rhinol 2018;8(12):1445–53.
29. Wallace D, Dykewicz M, Bernstein D, et al. The diagnosis and management of rhinitis: An updated practice parameter. J Allergy Clin Immunol 2008;122(2): S1–84.
30. Kaszuba SM, Baroody FM, deTineo M, et al. Superiority of an intranasal corticosteroid compared with an oral antihistamine in the as-needed treatment of seasonal allergic rhinitis. Arch Intern Med 2001;161(21):2581–7.
31. Brożek JL, Bousquet J, Agache I, et al. Allergic rhinitis and its impact on asthma (ARIA) guidelines—2016 revision. J Allergy Clin Immunol 2017;140(4):950–8.
32. Agnese C, Martone AM, Andrea P, et al. Anticholinergic drugs and negative outcomes in the older population: from biological plausibility to clinical evidence. Aging Clin Exp Res 2016;28(1):25–35.
33. Gray SL, Anderson ML, Dublin S, et al. Cumulative use of strong anticholinergics and incident dementia: a prospective cohort study. JAMA Intern Med 2015; 175(3):401–7.
34. Ousler GW, Wilcox KA, Gupta G, et al. An evaluation of the ocular drying effects of 2 systemic antihistamines: loratadine and cetirizine hydrochloride. Ann Allergy Asthma Immunol 2004;93(5):460–4.
35. Vacchiano C, Moore J, Rice GM, et al. Fexofenadine effects on cognitive performance in aviators at ground level and simulated altitude. Aviat Space Environ Med 2008;79(8):754–60.
36. Simons FER. Advances in H1-antihistamines. N Engl J Med 2004;351(21): 2203–17.
37. De Weck AL, Derer T, Bähre M. Investigation of the anti-allergic activity of azelastine on the immediate and late-phase reactions to allergens and histamine using telethermography. Clin Exp Allergy 2000;30(2):283–7.
38. Kaliner MA, Oppenheimer J, Farrar JR. Comprehensive review of olopatadine: the molecule and its clinical entities. Allergy Asthma Proc 2010;31(2):112–9.
39. Van Cauwenberge P, Bachert C, Passalacqua G, et al. Consensus statement on the treatment of allergic rhinitis. Allergy 2000;55(2):116–34.
40. Yáñez A, Rodrigo GJ. Intranasal corticosteroids versus topical H1 receptor antagonists for the treatment of allergic rhinitis: a systematic review with meta-analysis. Ann Allergy Asthma Immunol 2002;89(5):479–84.
41. Kaliner MA, Storms W, Tilles S, et al. Comparison of olopatadine 0.6% nasal spray versus fluticasone propionate 50 [micro]g in the treatment of seasonal allergic rhinitis. Allergy Asthma Proc 2009;30(3):255–62.
42. Ratner PH, Hampel F, Van Bavel J, et al. Combination therapy with azelastine hydrochloride nasal spray and fluticasone propionate nasal spray in the treatment of patients with seasonal allergic rhinitis. Ann Allergy Asthma Immunol 2008; 100(1):74–81.
43. Tietze KIN. Cromolyn sodium has limited use in self-management of allergic rhinitis. Pharm Today 2017;23(11):16.

44. Milgrom H, Biondi R, Georgitis JW, et al. Comparison of ipratropium bromide 0.03% with beclomethasone dipropionate in the treatment of perennial rhinitis in children. Ann Allergy Asthma Immunol 1999;83(2):105–11.

45. Nayak A, Langdon RB. Montelukast in the treatment of allergic rhinitis: an evidence-based review. Drugs 2007;67(6):887–901.

46. Wilson AM, O'Byrne PM, Parameswaran K. Leukotriene receptor antagonists for allergic rhinitis: a systematic review and meta-analysis. Am J Med 2004;116(5): 338–44.

47. Grainger J, Drake-Lee A. Montelukast in allergic rhinitis: a systematic review and meta-analysis. Clin Otolaryngol 2006;31(5):360–7.

48. Pullerits T, Praks L, Ristioja V, et al. Comparison of a nasal glucocorticoid, antileukotriene, and a combination of antileukotriene and antihistamine in the treatment of seasonal allergic rhinitis. J Allergy Clin Immunol 2002;109(6):949–55.

49. Lagos JA, Marshall GD. Montelukast in the management of allergic rhinitis. Ther Clin Risk Manag 2007;3(2):327–32.

50. Meltzer EO, Malmstrom K, Lu S, et al. Concomitant montelukast and loratadine as treatment for seasonal allergic rhinitis: a randomized, placebo-controlled clinical trial. J Allergy Clin Immunol 2000;105(5):917–22.

51. Cingi C, Gunhan K, Gage-White L, et al. Efficacy of leukotriene antagonists as concomitant therapy in allergic rhinitis. Laryngoscope 2010;120(9):1718–23.

52. Haarman MG, van Hunsel F, de Vries TW. Adverse drug reactions of montelukast in children and adults. Pharmacol Res Perspect 2017;5(5):e00341.

53. Department of Health and Human Services. Final Monograph for OTC Nasal Decongestant Drug Products; Final Rule. Fed Regist 1994;59. FR Doc No: 94-20456.

54. Baroody FM, Brown D, Gavanescu L, et al. Oxymetazoline adds to the effectiveness of fluticasone furoate in the treatment of perennial allergic rhinitis. J Allergy Clin Immunol 2011;127(4):927–34.

Management of Chronic Asthma in Adults

Huong Nguyen, DO, MS*, Munima Nasir, MD, FAAFP

KEYWORDS

- Chronic airway inflammation • Allergic • Non-allergic • Adult-onset
- Chronic asthma • Chronic management • Asthma in pregnancy • COVID-19

KEY POINTS

- Asthma can be diagnosed in childhood, or late-onset as an adult. Respiratory symptoms can present before 5 years of age, but it is often difficult to diagnose asthma in infants or toddlers.
- Respiratory symptoms, such as wheeze, shortness of breath, chest tightness, and cough vary over time and in intensity.
- Diagnosis is a combination of the history of symptoms along with bronchodilator reversibility testing.

INTRODUCTION

As defined by 2022 Global Initiative for Asthma (GINA): "Asthma is a heterogeneous disease, usually characterized by chronic airway inflammation. It is defined by the history of respiratory symptoms, such as wheeze, shortness of breath, chest tightness, and cough, that vary over time and in intensity, together with variable expiratory airflow limitation".[1]

Often, airway hyperresponsiveness, bronchoconstriction, and airway edema cause the reversible airway obstruction that is characteristic of asthma. One of the key drivers of asthma is acute and chronic inflammation.[2]

Asthma is a chronic respiratory disease that affects 1% to 18% of populations in varying countries.[1] As of 2017, asthma affects 25 million people, including 6 million children under the age of 18.[3] Although symptoms may resolve spontaneously, exacerbations can often be life-threatening and carry significant financial burdens to patients and the communities in which they live.

In the United States, asthma has a prevalence of 7.5% in children and 7.7% in adults.[4] In adults, women are more likely to die from asthma than men, whereas, in children, boys are more likely to die than girls.[5] This reversal of trends may be because

Family and Community Medicine, Penn State Health Milton S. Hershey Medical Center, 500 University Drive, H154/C1613, Hershey, PA, USA
* Corresponding author.
E-mail address: HNguyen10@pennstatehealth.psu.edu

Prim Care Clin Office Pract 50 (2023) 179–190
https://doi.org/10.1016/j.pop.2023.01.001
0095-4543/23/© 2023 Elsevier Inc. All rights reserved.

of the effects of testosterone on the lungs; testosterone has been found to decrease the swelling of airways in asthma, as suggested by some studies.[6] As of 2020, adults with asthma are five times more likely to die than children.[5] In the United States, black people are almost three times more likely to die from asthma than white people.[5] Deaths due to asthma were on the rise for the first time in over two decades in 2020; it is estimated that 11 people die in the United States from asthma every day.[5]

The annual economic cost of asthma, including medical costs and loss of work or school, was estimated to be over $81.9 billion; over $50.3 billion were due to medical costs.[7]

Clinical Presentation

- Asthmatics, particularly adults, will experience symptoms such as coughing, chest tightness, wheezing, or shortness of breath[1]
  - Often worse at night or early morning, and can vary in intensity and over time
  - Triggered by viral infections, exercise, allergen exposure, or changes in weather[8] (**Table 1**)

Risk factors for exacerbations of chronic asthma

- Poor asthma control[8–12]
- Poor adherence to chronic medications
- Incorrect use of inhaler/incorrect technique
- History of chronic sinusitis
- Chronic smoking

Diagnosing: criteria for asthma in adults

- There is no gold standard testing that is set for the diagnosis of asthma. Instead, diagnosis can be made by history, clinical findings, and observation of clinical course over time by a primary care provider, often a family physician. Objective measures, such as pulmonary function tests, can aid in the diagnosis, if this is available to the patient. Refer to **Table 2**.
- Pulmonary function may reveal expiratory airflow limitations and excessive variability in lung function.[1,13]

Table 1 Expected symptoms	
Respiratory Symptoms (Wheezing, Shortness of Breath, Cough, Chest Tightness) Typical of Asthma:	**Symptoms Unlikely Due to Asthma:**
Worse at night or when waking up	Isolated cough
Varies in intensity and time	Chronic sputum production
Symptoms triggered/worsened by viral infections, exercise, changes in weather, exercise	Chest pain
Symptoms can be worsened by laughter or strong smells (eg, perfume, incense, smoke, floral smells, car exhaust)	Exercise-induced dyspnea with noisy inspiration
	Shortness of breath along with paresthesia or light-headedness

Data from Levy ML, Fletcher M, Price DB, Hausend T, Halbert RJ, Yawn BP. International Primary Care Respiratory Group (IPCRG) guidelines: Diagnosis of respiratory diseases in primary care. Primary Care Respiratory Journal. 2006;15(1):20-34.

Table 2 Asthma categories of severity	
Intermittent	• Daytime symptoms ≤2 per week • ≤2 nocturnal awakenings per month • SABA to relieve symptoms ≤2 days per week • FEV1 measurements between exacerbations within normal range (≥80% of predicted) • FEV1/FVC ratio between exacerbations is normal (based on age-adjusted values) • ≤1 exacerbation requiring oral glucocorticoids per year
Mild persistent	• Symptoms >2 times weekly • Three to four nocturnal awakenings per month (fewer than every week) • SABA use for symptom relief >2 days out of the week (not daily) • Minor interference with normal activities • FEV1 measurements within normal range (≥80% of predicted)
Moderate persistent	• Daily symptoms • Nocturnal awakenings as often as once per week • Daily SABA for symptom relief. • Limitation in normal activity • FEV1 ≥60% and <80% of predicted and FEV1/FVC below normal
Severe persistent (defined by National Asthma Education and Prevention Program—NAEPP)	• Symptoms throughout the day • Nightly nocturnal awakening • Reliever medication needed for symptoms several times per day • Extreme limitations to daily activity

Abbreviation: SABA, short-acting beta-agonist.
Data from Refs.[19–22]

- ○ When the forced expiratory volume in the first second (FEV1) is reduced, confirm FEV1/forced vital capacity (FVC) is reduced.
  - ■ Lower limit of normal:
    - • Adults >0.75 to 0.80
    - • Children >0.90[14]
- ○ Diagnosis is better confirmed with greater variations in the variability of lung function testing, ie, if initial testing is normal, can consider repeating during the onset of symptoms or early in the morning
- • Partial (10%) reversibility of airflow obstruction on spirometry after beta2-agonist administration[2,15]
- • When a clinical diagnosis is not clear, perform a broncho-provocative challenge test with methacholine. A positive test is when the FEV1 decrease is more than 20% at 8 mg/mL.[2,16,17]
- • Monitoring test: peak flow meter[18]

Chronic Management and Maintenance

- • Main goals: optimize control of asthma symptoms and reduce risk of asthma exacerbations[1]
  - ○ Avoid allergens, air pollution, and other environmental triggers

- o Weight reduction
- o Smoking cessation
- Four essential components of management:
  - o Patient education
  - o Controlling asthma triggers
  - o Monitoring for changes in symptoms or lung function
  - o Pharmacologic therapy
- Patient–health care provider partnership[1]:
  - o Effective management should be a partnership between patient and health care provider[23]; shared decision-making has been shown to have improved outcomes[24,25]
  - o Education on self-management reduces morbidity in adults[23]

Treatment

- Treatment of asthma in the United States is guided by the Asthma Management Guidelines 2020, a report from the NAEPP Coordinating Committee Expert Panel Working Group by the National Heart, Lung, and Blood Institute (NHLBI) (**Fig. 1**).
- Treatment of asthma in Europe is guided by the GINA2022 (**Fig. 2**).
- With an initial diagnosis of asthma, it is important to initiate inhaled medications (see **Fig. 1**).
- Short-acting beta-agonists (SABA) for mild intermittent and persistent disease[20] (see **Fig. 1**).
  - o Intensity of treatment depends on the severity of symptoms
    - Intermittent asthma: typical use is every 4 to 6 hours, as needed
    - As prophylaxis: advise the patient to use 15 to 30 minutes before participating in physical activity
    - In severe exacerbations, as typically seen in the emergency room or in acute office visits: can use up to three treatments in 20-minute intervals as needed
    - Using SABA >2 times a week for relief of symptoms indicates poor control and requires treatment step up
- Inhaled maintenance therapies for persistent disease[20] (see **Fig. 1**)
  - o Inhaled maintenance therapies are the mainstay of management for mild persistent, moderate to severe, and uncontrolled persistent asthmatics.
- Biologics for severe persistent disease
  - o Anti-IgE: consider in allergic-driven disease
    - Omalizumab injections every 2 to 4 weeks: consider when serum IgE levels are between 30 and 700.
    - Mechanism of action: binds to third constant domain of IgE heavy chains and forms complexes with free IgE, preventing interaction with these receptors on mast cells and basophils
    - Minimum of 12 weeks of treatment to determine the efficacy
    - Adverse effects: hypersensitity including anaphylaxis, urticaria, and injection site reactions
  - o Anti-IL5: consider when there are high serum eosinophils
    - Mepolizumab injections once every 4 weeks: consider: when eosinophil levels >150.
      Mechanism of action: inhibits IL-5 signaling and reduces the production of eosinophils
      Adverse effects: injection site reactions, headache, and hypersensitivity reactions

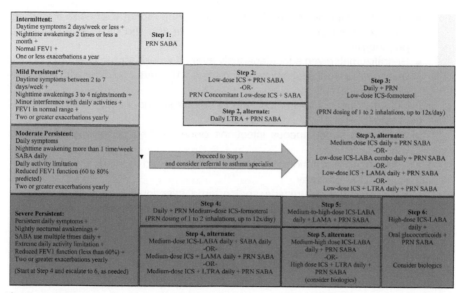

Fig. 1. Assessment and treatment of asthma in ages 12 years and older as defined by the National Asthma Education and Prevention Program: Expert Panel Working Group 2020. ICS, inhaled corticosteroids; LABA, long-acting beta-agonist; LAMA, long-acting muscarinic antagonist; LTRA, leukotriene receptor antagonist; PRN, as needed; SABA, short-acting beta-agonist. [a]If poorly controlled Mild Persistent Asthma, proceed to Step 3. (*Adapted from* Expert Panel Working Group of the National Heart, Lung, and Blood Institute (NHLBI) administered and coordinated National Asthma Education and Prevention Program Coordinating Committee (NAEPPCC); Cloutier MM, Baptist AP, Blake KV, Brooks EG, Bryant-Stephens T, DiMango E, Dixon AE, Elward KS, Hartert T, Krishnan JA, Lemanske RF Jr, Ouellette DR, Pace WD, Schatz M, Skolnik NS, Stout JW, Teach SJ, Umscheid CA, Walsh CG. 2020 Focused Updates to the Asthma Management Guidelines: A Report from the National Asthma Education and Prevention Program Coordinating Committee Expert Panel Working Group. J Allergy Clin Immunol. 2020 Dec;146(6):1217-1270. https://doi.org/10.1016/j.jaci.2020.10.003. Erratum in: J Allergy Clin Immunol. 2021 Apr;147(4):1528-1530. PMID: 33280709; PMCID: PMC7924476.)

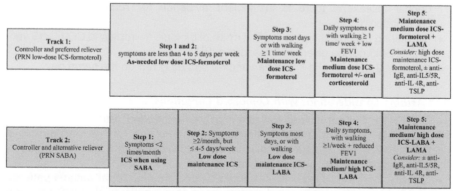

Fig. 2. Assessment and treatment of asthma as defined by GINA 2022. PRN, as needed; TSLP, thymic stromal lymphopoietin. (*Data from* Global Strategy for Asthma Management and Prevention. Global Initiative for Asthma. Updated 2022. Accessed July 1, 2022. https://ginasthma.org/wp-content/uploads/2022/07/GINA-Main-Report-2022-FINAL-22-07-02-WMS.pdf (1) (1) (1).)

- Reslizumab infusions over 20 to 50 minutes, 3 mg/kg every 4 to 6 months; consider in severe asthmatics >18 years of age and have an eosinophilic phenotype
- Benralizumab given subcutaneously every 4 weeks for the first three doses, then every 8 weeks for severe asthmatics >12 years and older with an eosinophilic predominance
  ○ Anti-IL4/IL13: consider in moderate to severe eosinophilic or oral glucocorticoid dependent
    - Dupilumab subcutaneous injections once (loading dose) and then every other week
      • Mechanism of action: binds to IL-4 receptor and modifies signaling of IL-4 and IL-13 pathway
      • Adverse effects: urticaria, angioedema, injection site rash, erythema multiforme, serum sickness-like reaction, conjunctivitis, blepharitis, keratitis, eye pruritis, xerophthalmia
- Consider consulting an asthma specialist if the patient is experiencing uncontrolled moderate persistent asthma, or if the patient is requiring Step 3 of treatment. If the patient has severe persistent asthma, that is, requiring Step 4 of treatment, consult an asthma specialist (see **Fig. 1**).
- Control assessment:
  ○ First check: Adherence, correct inhaler technique, environmental factors, comorbid conditions
  ○ Escalate treatment if not controlled; can reassess in 2 to 6 weeks
  ○ Deescalate treatment if asthma has been well controlled for at least 3 months consecutively
- Vitamin D: In patients who require systemic corticosteroids, vitamin D supplementation may reduce the rate of exacerbation in patients with baseline 25(OH)D of less than 25 to 30 nmol/L.[26,27] Overall, current studies are not of good quality, and more studies are needed for clear recommendations.[1]

Vaccine Recommendations

- Annual influenza vaccine[1,28]
- Although children and the elderly who have asthma are more at risk of pneumococcal disease,[29] there is insufficient evidence for routine pneumococcal vaccination[30]
- If requiring biologic therapy, the first dose of biologic therapy and COVID-19 vaccine should not be given on the same day[1]
- COVID-19 vaccine and influenza vaccine can be given on the same day[1]

Adult Asthma Considerations with Comorbid Conditions

- COVID-19: Current studies indicate that well-controlled asthmatics are not at increased risk of COVID-19-related death; There is an increased risk of COVID-19 death in asthmatics who recently needed oral corticosteroids or were hospitalized for severe asthma.[1]
- Obesity: Body mass index (BMI) should be documented for all asthma patients, as it is more difficult to control symptoms in obese patients.[31–34] ICS are a key treatment of asthma in obese patients. However, the clinical response to glucocorticoid-containing regimens is reduced in asthmatics who are overweight or obese.[34] Improved quality of life and control of asthma symptoms are seen with 5% to 10% weight reduction.[35]

- Gastroesophageal reflux disease (GERD): Symptoms are more common in asthmatics than in the general population.[36] Treatment with proton pump inhibitors (PPI) in patients who have both asthma and GERD has a small benefit for lung function; PPI therapy in adult asthmatics yields a small improvement in morning peak expiratory flow.[37,38] However, there is still limited data that are statistically significant to recommend empirical PPI use in the routine treatment of asthma.[37]

Asthma in Pregnancy

- Exacerbations are common and typically occur in the second trimester.[39]
- Poorly controlled asthma can result in worse outcomes for the baby (pre-term delivery, low birth weight) and the mother (pre-eclampsia). Well-controlled asthma during pregnancy has little or no increased risk of adverse maternal or fetal complications.[40]
- ICS, beta2-agonists, montelukast, or theophylline are not associated with increased incidence of fetal abnormalities[41]
  - Use of ICS reduces the risk of having asthma exacerbations during pregnancy[11,40,42]
- Important to aggressively treat acute exacerbations of asthma with SABA, oxygen, and administration of systemic corticosteroids to prevent fetal hypoxia[1]
- During labor and delivery: continue usual controller medications and add reliever when needed. If acute exacerbation during delivery, manage with SABA.[1]
  - If high doses of beta-agonist are given within 48 hours before delivery, neonatal hypoglycemia should be monitored with blood glucose checks for the first 24 hours.[43,44]

DISCUSSION

In the United States, asthma is a common disease affecting approximately 25 million people, of which 20 million are adults aged 18 and older.[2] As of 2018, asthma accounted for 1.6 million emergency department visits, 178,530 inpatient hospitalizations,[45,46] and 5.8 million office visits.[4] Although treatment is widely available, and the ability to diagnose asthma by clinical judgment and testing has improved drastically, deaths caused by asthma or asthma exacerbations remain prominent. For the first time in 20 years, deaths due to asthma were on the rise, with 4,145 people dying from complications from asthma; proper treatment and care could have prevented nearly all these deaths.[5] Although ICS may control symptoms, it alone does not change the underlying disease process or progression of asthma.[47] Thus, it is important to provide appropriate medications to manage and control chronic asthma and to identify and treat immediate exacerbations. Medications containing ICS are considered controller medications and are used to reduce airway inflammation, control asthma symptoms, and reduce asthma exacerbations.[48]

Although long-term studies of COVID-19 are currently limited, studies to date suggest that well-controlled asthmatics are not at risk of COVID-19-related deaths.[49,50] However, in severe asthmatics requiring hospitalization[51] and asthmatics requiring oral corticosteroids to control acute exacerbations,[49,52] the risk of COVID-19-related death was increased.

Since 2007, the NHLBI has made substantial changes in recommendations in the most recent 2020 guidelines, to include changes regarding allergen mitigation, ICS use, and immunotherapy. Regarding treatment in asthmatics ages 12 and older with mild persistent asthma, a conditional recommendation of treatment now includes concomitant as-needed ICS and SABA use versus daily low-dose ICS and SABA as needed for quick relief. A strong recommendation in the 2020 guidelines for asthmatics ages 4 years and older with moderate to severe persistent asthma includes starting treatment with ICS-formoterol in a single inhaler as both a daily controller and reliever therapy.[20] SMART therapy, or "single maintenance and reliever therapy," is perhaps the most impactful recommendation from the 2020 guideline. The NHLBI recommends the daily use of ICS–LABA combinations that contain formoterol be initiated in moderate persistent asthma. With proper use, SMART therapy was found to significantly reduce asthma exacerbations, emergency room visits, hospitalizations, as well as significantly lower the need for systemic corticosteroids.[20,53–56]

Although treatment is often aimed at symptom control, severe asthmatics can often remain uncontrolled despite the use and adherence to high-dose controller therapy. Over the last few decades, biologic drugs have been developed to target specific causative mechanisms that have allowed asthma treatment to be personalized.[57,58] Approval by the United States Food and Drug Administration for biologics, beginning with omalizumab in 2003, has allowed for substantial clinical studies to evaluate the efficacy of treatment in uncontrolled severe asthmatics. Biologics that are currently available, including omalizumab, mepolizumab, reslizumab, and benralizumab have been shown to be effective in reduction of asthma exacerbations, systemic corticosteroid treatment, and overall improvement of lung function and quality of life in severe asthmatics.[59,60]

As per the 2022 GINA guidelines, two types of reliever medications can be prescribed to asthmatics: an as-needed low-dose ICS-formoterol or an as-needed SABA, refer to **Fig. 2**. When considering between the rescue medications, the use of SABA daily increases the risk of asthma exacerbations, and therefore, ICS budesonide-formoterol is the preferred rescue medication.[61,62] An important goal in asthma management is reducing and eventually eliminating the need for SABA relievers.[1] Although the GINA guidelines are used in Europe, they are not followed in the United States.

Primary care physicians are often the first providers to recognize, diagnose, and treat patients with asthma. It is evident that physicians must communicate with patients the importance of taking their prescribed asthma medications, avoidance of triggers, as well as supporting and encouraging patients to take ownership of their chronic regimen. It is important to treat asthmatics by prescribing the correct medications and inhalers to control chronic asthma. It is also crucial for physicians to recognize and immediately treat acute exacerbations to prevent avoidable complications, including hospitalizations, missed days at work or school, or even death. Primary care physicians must be able to recognize when asthma symptoms are not well controlled and require higher care, particularly when requiring the addition of biologics. It is at this step in management that referral to an asthma specialist, a pulmonologist, or an allergist, is crucial for appropriate care. The ability to do this will aid in the reduction of the general economic burden, but perhaps more importantly, it ultimately reduces the economic and physical burden on patients.

CLINICS CARE POINTS

- When evaluating adolescent asthmatics, do it in private without a parent or guardian to obtain accurate information to adequately diagnose the severity and correct treatment.
- In pregnant asthmatics, continue controller medications and add reliever medications during labor and delivery. Although rare, if there is an acute exacerbation during delivery, administer SABA.

> - Well-controlled asthmatics are not at an increased risk of COVID-19-related deaths.
> - There is insufficient evidence for routine pneumococcal vaccination in asthmatics who are young or elderly.

DISCLOSURE

The authors have no financial conflicts of interest to disclose.

REFERENCES

1. Global Strategy for Asthma Management and Prevention. Global Initiative for Asthma. 2022. Available at: https://ginasthma.org/wp-content/uploads/2022/07/GINA-Main-Report-2022-FINAL-22-07-02-WMS.pdf. Accessed July 1, 2022.
2. Partin M, Morrison A, Carter M, et al. Asthma (chronic management). In: Ebell M, French L, Slawson D, editors. Essential evidence plus. Wiley Subscription Services; 2022.
3. 2019 National Health Interview Survey (NHIS) data. Centers for Disease Control and Prevention. Available at: https://www.cdc.gov/asthma/nhis/2019/data.htm. Accessed July 19, 2022.
4. National Ambulatory Medical Care Survey: 2018 national summary. 2021. Available at: https://www.cdc.gov/nchs/data/ahcd/namcs_summary/2018-namcs-web-tables-508.pdf. Accessed July 17, 2022.
5. National Vital Statistics System: Mortality (1999-2018). Available at: https://wonder.cdc.gov/ucd-icd10.html. Accessed July 19, 2022.
6. Fuseini H, Newcomb DC. Mechanisms driving gender differences in asthma. Curr Allergy Asthma Rep 2017;17(3). https://doi.org/10.1007/s11882-017-0686-1.
7. Nurmagambetov T, Kuwahara R, Garbe P. The economic burden of asthma in the United States, 2008–2013. Annals of the American Thoracic Society 2018;15(3): 348–56.
8. Loymans RJ, Honkoop PJ, Termeer EH, et al. Identifying patients at risk for severe exacerbations of asthma: development and external validation of a multivariable prediction model. Thorax 2016;71(9):838–46.
9. McCoy K, Shade D, Irvin C, et al. Predicting episodes of poor asthma control in treated patients with asthma. J Allergy Clin Immunol 2006;118(6):1226–33.
10. Meltzer EO, Busse WW, Wenzel SE, et al. Use of the asthma control questionnaire to predict future risk of asthma exacerbation. J Allergy Clin Immunol 2011;127(1): 167–72.
11. Schatz M, Zeiger RS, Yang S-J, et al. The relationship of asthma impairment determined by psychometric tools to future asthma exacerbations. Chest 2012; 141(1):66–72.
12. Levy ML, Fletcher M, Price DB, et al. International Primary Care Respiratory Group (IPCRG) guidelines: Diagnosis of respiratory diseases in primary care. Prim Care Respir J 2006;15(1):20–34.
13. Smith AD, Cowan JO, Filsell S, et al. Diagnosing asthma: Comparisons between exhaled nitric oxide measurements and conventional tests. Am J Respir Crit Care Med 2004;169(4):473–8.
14. Quanjer PH, Stanojevic S, Cole TJ, et al. Multi-ethnic reference values for spirometry for the 3–95-yr age range: The Global Lung Function 2012 equations. Eur Respir J 2012;40(6):1324–43.

15. Pellegrino R. Interpretative strategies for lung function tests. Eur Respir J 2005; 26(5):948–68.
16. Crapo RO, Casaburi R, Coates AL, et al. Guidelines for methacholine and exercise challenge testing—1999. Am J Respir Crit Care Med 2000;161(1):309–29.
17. Hunter CJ, Brightling CE, Woltmann G, et al. A comparison of the validity of different diagnostic tests in adults with asthma. Chest 2002;121(4):1051–7.
18. McCoy EK, Thomas JL, Sowell RS, et al. An evaluation of peak expiratory flow monitoring: A comparison of sitting versus standing measurements. J Am Board Fam Med 2010;23(2):166–70.
19. Chung KF, Wenzel SE, Brozek JL. Comment on: International ERS/ATS guidelines on definition, evaluation and treatment of severe asthma. Eur Respir J 2014;43: 343–73.
20. 2020 Focused Updates to the Asthma Management Guidelines. National Heart, Lung, and Blood Institute. 2021. Available at: https://www.nhlbi.nih.gov/resources/2020-focused-updates-asthma-management-guidelines. Accessed July 1, 2022.
21. Taylor DR, Bateman ED, Boulet L-P, et al. A new perspective on concepts of asthma severity and control. Eur Respir J 2008;32(3):545–54.
22. Cloutier MM, Baptist AP, Blake KV, et al. 2020 focused updates to the Asthma Management Guidelines: A report from the National Asthma Education and Prevention Program Coordinating Committee Expert Panel Working Group. J Allergy Clin Immunol 2020;146(6):1217–70.
23. Gibson PG, Powell H, Wilson A, et al. Self-management education and regular practitioner review for adults with asthma. Cochrane Database Syst Rev 2003. https://doi.org/10.1002/14651858.cd001117.
24. Wilson SR, Strub P, Buist AS, et al. Shared treatment decision making improves adherence and outcomes in poorly controlled asthma. Am J Respir Crit Care Med 2010;181(6):566–77.
25. Guevara JP. Effects of educational interventions for self management of asthma in children and adolescents: Systematic review and meta-analysis. BMJ 2003; 326(7402):1308.
26. Jolliffe DA, Greenberg L, Hooper RL, et al. Vitamin D supplementation to prevent Asthma Exacerbations: a systematic review and meta-analysis of individual participant data. Lancet Respir Med 2017;5(11):881–90.
27. Andújar-Espinosa R, Salinero-González L, Illán-Gómez F, et al. Effect of vitamin D supplementation on asthma control in patients with vitamin D deficiency: the ACVID randomised clinical trial. Thorax 2020;76(2):126–33.
28. Vasileiou E, Sheikh A, Butler C, et al. Effectiveness of influenza vaccines in asthma: a systematic review and meta-analysis. Clin Infect Dis 2017;65(8): 1388–95.
29. Li L, Cheng Y, Tu X, et al. Association between asthma and invasive pneumococcal disease risk: a systematic review and meta-analysis. Allergy Asthma Clin Immunol 2020;16(1). https://doi.org/10.1186/s13223-020-00492-4.
30. Sheikh A, Alves B, Dhami S. Pneumococcal vaccine for asthma. Cochrane Database Syst Rev 2002;2014(6). https://doi.org/10.1002/14651858.cd002165.
31. Boulet L-P. Asthma and obesity. Clin Exp Allergy 2012;43(1):8–21.
32. Lavoie KL, Bacon SL, Labrecque M, et al. Higher BMI is associated with worse asthma control and quality of life but not asthma severity. Respir Med 2006; 100(4):648–57.
33. Saint-Pierre P, Bourdin A, Chanez P, et al. Are overweight asthmatics more difficult to control? Allergy 2006;61:79–84.

34. Sutherland ER, Goleva E, Strand M, et al. Body mass and glucocorticoid response in asthma. Am J Respir Crit Care Med 2008;178(7):682–7.

35. Scott HA, Gibson PG, Garg ML, et al. Dietary restriction and exercise improve airway inflammation and clinical outcomes in overweight and obese asthma: A randomized trial. Clin Exp Allergy 2012;43(1):36–49.

36. Boulet L-P. Influence of comorbid conditions on asthma. Eur Respir J 2009;33(4): 897–906.

37. Chan WW, Chiou E, Obstein KL, et al. The efficacy of proton pump inhibitors for the treatment of asthma in adults. Arch Intern Med 2011;171(7):620–9.

38. Kopsaftis Z, Yap HS, Tin KS, et al. Pharmacological and surgical interventions for the treatment of gastro-oesophageal reflux in adults and children with asthma. Cochrane Database Syst Rev 2021;2021(5). https://doi.org/10.1002/14651858. cd001496.

39. Murphy VE, Clifton VL, Gibson PG. Asthma exacerbations during pregnancy: Incidence and association with adverse pregnancy outcomes. Thorax 2006; 61(2):169–76.

40. Murphy VE, Gibson PG. Asthma in pregnancy. Clin Chest Med 2011;32(1): 93–110.

41. Lim A, Stewart K, König K, et al. Systematic review of the safety of regular preventive asthma medications during pregnancy. Ann Pharmacother 2011;45(7–8): 931–45.

42. Wendel PJ, Ramin SM, Barnett-Hamm C, et al. Asthma treatment in pregnancy: A randomized controlled study. Am J Obstet Gynecol 1996;175(1):150–4.

43. Nelson-Piercy C. Respiratory diseases in pregnancy bullet 1: asthma in pregnancy. Thorax 2001;56(4):325–8.

44. Patton GC, Viner R. Pubertal transitions in health. Lancet 2007;369:1130–9.

45. Healthcare Cost and Utilization Project (2018). 2022. Available at: http://www. cdc.gov/asthma/national-surveillance-data/healthcare-use.htm. Accessed July 20, 2022.

46. National Hospital Ambulatory Medical Care Survey (2010-2018). National Center for Health Statistics. 2022. Available at: https://www.cdc.gov/asthma/national-surveillance-data/healthcare-use.htm. Accessed July 20, 2022.

47. Guilbert TW, Morgan WJ, Zeiger RS, et al. Long-term inhaled corticosteroids in preschool children at high risk for asthma. N Engl J Med 2006;354(19):1985–97.

48. O'Byrne PM, Pedersen S, Lamm CJ, et al. Severe exacerbations and decline in lung function in asthma. Am J Respir Crit Care Med 2009;179(1):19–24.

49. Williamson EJ, Walker AJ, Bhaskaran K, et al. Factors associated with covid-19-related death using OpenSAFELY. Nature 2020;584(7821):430–6.

50. Liu S, Cao Y, Du T, et al. Prevalence of comorbid asthma and related outcomes in COVID-19: a systematic review and meta-analysis. J Allergy Clin Immunol Pract 2021;9(2):693–701.

51. Bloom CI, Drake TM, Docherty AB, et al. Risk of adverse outcomes in patients with underlying respiratory conditions admitted to hospital with covid-19: A national, multicentre prospective cohort study using the ISARIC who clinical characterisation protocol UK. Lancet Respir Med 2021. https://doi.org/10.1016/ s2213-2600(21)00013-8.

52. Shi T, Pan J, Katikireddi SV, et al. Risk of COVID-19 hospital admission among children aged 5–17 years with asthma in Scotland: A national incident cohort study. Lancet Respir Med 2022;10(2):191–8.

53. O'Byrne PM, Bisgaard H, Godard PP, et al. Budesonide/formoterol combination therapy as both maintenance and reliever medication in asthma. Am J Respir Crit Care Med 2005;171(2):129–36.

54. Atienza T, Aquino T, Fernandez M, et al. Budesonide/formoterol maintenance and reliever therapy via Turbuhaler versus fixed-dose budesonide/formoterol plus terbutaline in patients with asthma: Phase III study results. Respirology 2013;18(2): 354–63.

55. Papi A, Corradi M, Pigeon-Francisco C, et al. Beclometasone–Formoterol as maintenance and reliever treatment in patients with asthma: a double-blind, randomised controlled trial. Lancet Respir Med 2013;1(1):23–31.

56. Vogelmeier C, Boutet S, Merino JM, et al. Budesonide/Formoterol Maintenance and reliever therapy: An effective asthma treatment option? Eur Respir J 2005; 26(6):1191. EUR RESPIR J 2005; 26: 819-828.

57. Paoletti G, Pepys J, Casini M, et al. Biologics in severe asthma: The role of real-world evidence from registries. Eur Respir Rev 2022;31(164):210278.

58. Ferrando M, Bagnasco D, Heffler E, et al. Personalizing the approach to asthma treatment. Expert Review of Precision Medicine and Drug Development 2018; 3(5):299–304.

59. Solèr M, Matz J, Townley R, et al. The anti-ige antibody omalizumab reduces exacerbations and steroid requirement in allergic asthmatics. Eur Respir J 2001; 18(2):254–61.

60. Fahy JV, Fleming HE, Wong HH, et al. The effect of an anti-ige monoclonal antibody on the early- and late-phase responses to allergen inhalation in asthmatic subjects. Am J Respir Crit Care Med 1997;155(6):1828–34.

61. Nwaru BI, Ekström M, Hasvold P, et al. Overuse of short-acting β2-agonists in asthma is associated with increased risk of exacerbation and mortality: A nationwide cohort study of the global sabina programme. Eur Respir J 2020;55(4): 1901872.

62. Raissy HH, Kelly HW, Harkins M, et al. Inhaled corticosteroids in lung diseases. Am J Respir Crit Care Med 2013;187(8):798–803.

Atopic Dermatitis

Karl T. Clebak, MD, MHA[a],*, Leesha Helm, MD, MPH[a],
Prabhdeep Uppal, DO, MS[b,c,1], Christopher R. Davis, MD, MPH[a],
Matthew F. Helm, MD[d]

KEYWORDS

- Atopic dermatitis • Emollients and skin care • Topical therapy • Systemic therapy
- Phototherapy

KEY POINTS

- Atopic dermatitis (AD) is a common, chronic relapsing, and remitting inflammatory skin disease that is characterized by erythematous, scaly, and pruritic lesions often located over the flexural surfaces.
- Good skin hygiene and the use of emollients are recommended for chronic treatment in all patients with AD.
- Topical corticosteroids are first-line treatments during AD exacerbations.
- Systemic therapies including monoclonal antibody treatments and phototherapy are effective in patients with moderate-to-severe AD not responsive to topical therapies.

INTRODUCTION

Atopic dermatitis (AD), also known as atopic eczema, is a chronic relapsing inflammatory skin disease that is characterized by erythematous, scaly, and pruritic lesions often located over the flexural surfaces in adults (**Fig. 1**).[1] In infants, the lesions predominantly affect the face, scalp, trunk, and extensor surfaces. Acutely, the lesions are vesicular with open weeping and crusting eruption. In the subacute phase, the lesions present as scaly and dry fissures, which over time are lichenified from repeated scratching. Another feature of chronic AD is decreased erythema compared with the acute state.[1] AD is often associated with atopic conditions, such as allergies and asthma. In addition to the association with closely related atopic conditions, AD is related to other diseases such as obesity, cardiovascular disease, and psychological diseases such as anxiety and depression.[2,3]

[a] Department of Family and Community Medicine, Penn State Health Milton. S Hershey Medical Center, 500 University Drive, H154/C1613 Hershey, PA 17033, USA; [b] Department of Family and Community Medicine, ChristianaCare, 1401 Foulk Road, Suite 100B, Wilmington, DE 19803, USA; [c] Department of Emergency Medicine, ChristianaCare, 1401 Foulk Road, Suite 100B, Wilmington, DE 19803, USA; [d] Department of Dermatology, Penn State Health Milton. S Hershey Medical Center, 500 University Drive, Suite 4300, MC HU14, Hershey, PA 17033, USA
[1] Present address: 4755 Ogletown-Stanton Road, Newark, DE 19718, USA
* Corresponding author. 500 University Drive, H154/C1613, Hershey, PA 17033.
E-mail address: Kclebak@pennstatehealth.psu.edu

Prim Care Clin Office Pract 50 (2023) 191–203
https://doi.org/10.1016/j.pop.2022.12.004
0095-4543/23/© 2022 Elsevier Inc. All rights reserved.

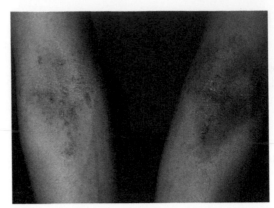

Fig. 1. Atopic dermatitis: pink scaly papules and plaques in the antecubital fossa.

Multiple theories exist regarding the pathophysiology of AD and include a complex interplay of factors including genetics, the immune system, the environment, and the skin surface microbiome. Two major theories exist to explain the pathophysiology of AD: the inside-out and outside-in hypotheses. The inside-out hypothesis suggests inflammation or dysregulation of the immune system creates skin barrier defects that further allow penetration of allergens and irritants.[2,3] The outside-in hypothesis suggests that epidermal skin barrier impairments lead to immune dysregulation and allergic sensitization.[4]

Both innate and acquired immune responses have a role in the pathogenesis of AD. The Th2 response is further exacerbated by Langerhans cells in the epidermis, which are specialized immune cells that have a heightened response to allergen and irritant antigens. Implicated cytokines in this causal pathway include IL-4, IL-13, IL-31, and IL-22 many of which are targeted by new biologic medications.[5,6] IL-31 has specifically been shown to be important in the pathogenesis of pruritus. This itch–scratch cycle ultimately worsens the inflammation of AD by decreasing filaggrin (FLG), ceramides, and antimicrobial peptides while increasing bacterial colonization and infections of the skin, which become difficult to control.

The pathogenesis of AD involves skin barrier dysfunction, often times triggered by FLG mutations. Emerging evidence shows that disorder in FLG expression plays a critical role in developing AD. FLG are proteins that bind keratin in epidermal cells. Loss of FLG leads to flattening of skin surface cells, a decrease in natural moisturizing factors of the skin, and an increase in skin pH, which leads to increased activity of proteases and enzymes that break down proteins that hold skin epidermal cells together and ultimately cytokines that promote skin inflammation.[6–8]

Other factors to consider that contribute to the process of inflammation include the skin microbiome, viral, bacterial, and fungal infections, stress, climate, food, and environmental allergens.[6]

OBSERVATION/ASSESSMENT/EVALUATION

The 3 phases of AD are infantile, childhood, and adult.

Infantile Atopic Dermatitis

Clinical presentation and differential diagnosis
Infantile AD typically manifests from birth to 2 years and is part of a multitude of allergic conditions that develop during infancy known as "atopic march." This progressive

atopy begins with the development of AD and subsequently allergic rhinitis and asthma in later childhood. Infants typically present with erythematous papules and vesicles seen on the cheeks, forehead, or scalp. In infants, atopic lesions often involve the face, scalp, and extensor surfaces (as opposed to adult AD), and the affected areas can have serous oozing and crusting (**Fig. 2**). The diaper area is often spared due to moisture retention of the diaper.[9]

Diagnosis and classification

The "Hanifin and Rajka" criteria and the UK Working Party's Diagnostic Criteria for Atopic Dermatitis are the most widely cited criteria used.[10–13]

Five major clinical features based on these criteria are (4 required for diagnosis) as follows:

1. pruritus
2. a chronic, relapsing course
3. typical distribution
4. family or personal history of atopy
5. onset before 2 years of age.

Minor criteria are also frequently observed and include the following:

- Early age of onset
- Xerosis
- Palmar hyperlinearity, ichthyosis, keratosis pilaris
- Immediate skin test reactivity, elevated serum IgE
- Cutaneous infection, including *Staphylococcus aureus* and Herpes simplex virus
- Nipple eczema
- Cheilitis
- Pityriasis alba
- White dermatographism, delayed blanching
- Perifollicular accentuation
- Anterior subcapsular cataracts
- Itch when sweating
- Nonspecific hand or foot dermatitis
- Recurrent conjunctivitis
- Dennie-Morgan folds
- Keratoconus

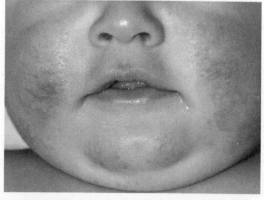

Fig. 2. Infantile atopic dermatitis: pink oozing vesicles on the cheeks.

- Facial erythema or pallor

Scoring tools to measure disease severity such as the Severity Scoring of Atopic Dermatitis index and the Eczema Area and Severity index can be used for research and clinical practice. It is also important to note that infantile AD affects quality of life not just for the patient but also for the parent and caretaker. Infants often have intense pruritus and sleep disturbances, and parents or caretakers are often affected by the cost of medication, poor sleep, time off of work, and emotional stress because of their care for their child with AD.[9]

Management

Treatment of infantile AD includes topical emollients and corticosteroids. Emollients improve skin hydration and have been shown to decrease the number of flares. There is little evidence to show whether certain emollients are superior to others but ideally should be free of sensitizing agents. First-line medication option in the management of AD is topical corticosteroids (TCS), which are classified into 7 groups based on potency. Low-potency TCS should be used for long-term management because children are more prone to develop side effects. Because infants have thinner skin and a larger surface-area-to-weight ratio, they are likely to absorb increased amounts of the medication compared with adults. Commonly used TCS approved for infants aged 3 months and older include low-to-medium potency TCS such as desonide, fluocinolone acetonide oil, hydrocortisone butyrate, or triamcinolone. Ointment is based in petrolatum and is more effective at healing the skin than lotions or creams that are water based. Current treatment guidelines do not recommend more than twice-daily application of TCS. Side effects include skin atrophy, striae, acne, and telangiectasia. For this reason, they should be used for the shortest duration needed to control the flare-up and on an as-needed basis after that.

Topical calcineurin inhibitors such as tacrolimus and pimecrolimus are second-line treatment options. These nonsteroidal medications inhibit calcineurin in the skin, blocking T-cell activation, and the release of cytokines. They are approved in the United States by the Food and Drug Administration for children aged 2 years and older and are usually used in conjunction with TCS. Adverse effects include skin burning and irritation, so patients should be counseled on using sun protection.[9]

Wet wrap therapy is a useful technique to treat persistent and refractory AD. They are best done in the evening before bed where a topical steroid is placed on eczematous lesions, a moist dressing is placed over the lesion and then a dry one on top of that. Then the patient puts on their clothing and leaves them on for several hours over night. Results are quite remarkable even after a few days using this method.

Importantly, peanut introduction should not be delayed in children simply due to the presence of AD. The Learning Early about Peanut Allergy trial examined the introduction of peanuts in infants with severe AD or egg allergy, and concluded that early and sustained peanut consumption in this group resulted in notably lower rates of peanut allergy at 60 months of age.[14] In 2017, the National Institute of Allergy and Infectious Diseases developed an addendum of guidelines specifically to address the prevention of peanut allergy for infants at various risk levels[15] (**Table 1**).

Toddler and School Age Atopic Dermatitis

The distribution of dermatitis changes as children age. From age 2 to 12 years, with walking, flexural surface involvement (antecubital fossae, popliteal fossae, neck, wrists, and ankles) is often seen. With eating and drooling, dermatitis can spread to the mouth and chin. Lichenification due to chronicity of symptoms and scratching also occurs. Although during the school years, AD will improve, the function of the

Table 1
Summary of addendum guidelines for the prevention of peanut allergy

Infant Criteria	Recommendations	Earliest Age of Peanut Introduction
Severe eczema, egg allergy, or both	Strongly consider evaluation with peanut-specific IgE and/or skin prick test and, if necessary, an oral food challenge. Based on test results, introduce peanut-containing foods	4–6 mo
Mild-to-moderate eczema	Introduce peanut-containing foods	Around 6 mo
No eczema or any food allergy	Introduce peanut-containing foods	Age-appropriate and in accordance with family preferences and cultural practices

From Togias A, Cooper SF, Acebal ML, Assa'ad A, Baker JR Jr, Beck LA, Block J, Byrd-Bredbenner C, Chan ES, Eichenfield LF, Fleischer DM, Fuchs GJ 3rd, Furuta GT, Greenhawt MJ, Gupta RS, Habich M, Jones SM, Keaton K, Muraro A, Plaut M, Rosenwasser LJ, Rotrosen D, Sampson HA, Schneider LC, Sicherer SH, Sidbury R, Spergel J, Stukus DR, Venter C, Boyce JA. Addendum guidelines for the prevention of peanut allergy in the United States: Report of the National Institute of Allergy and Infectious Diseases-sponsored expert panel. J Allergy Clin Immunol. 2017 Jan;139(1):29-44.

skin barrier will never be normal. The differential for manifestations of AD in this age group includes discoid eczema, pityriasis alba, and lip licker's dermatitis.[16]

Clinical presentation and differential diagnosis
Similar diagnosis strategies to that used for infantile AD can be used. See guidelines and therapeutics table for specific age-based options for treatment.

Adult Atopic Dermatitis

There is a variety of presentations of the adult phase. The flexural pattern can persist and is common or become more diffuse. Some adults who had complete resolution of AD as a child, may develop hand dermatitis due to occupational exposures. The upper eyelids and lips are other frequent affected areas in adults. Denni-Morgan folds, or a fold of skin under the lower eyelids, can be seen when chronic eyelid dermatitis develops. Dry skin, white dermographism, hyperlinear palms, ichthyosis vulgaris, and keratosis pilaris are common associated manifestations of AD in adults. Lichenification and fissuring can commonly occur with chronicity (**Figs. 3** and **4**) Adult-onset dermatitis also can occur but is unusual.[17]

Scoring tools used now to assess disease severity in patients with skin of color can underestimate the severity of disease due to erythema in adult AD in skin of color being violaceous. Postinflammatory hypopigmentation and hyperpigmentation occur more commonly in skin of color and is often a source of distress (**Fig. 5**). With scratching and rubbing, patients with skin of color can also more commonly develop lichen simplex or nodular prurigo.[18]

Similar diagnosis strategies to that used for infantile AD can be used. See the guidelines and therapeutics table below for specific age-based options for treatment.

PREVALENCE/INCIDENCE

AD affects 10% to 20% of the population in developed countries.[19] It is ranked as the third most prevalent dermatologic condition but was the greatest contributor to

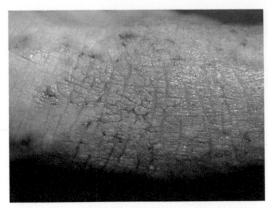

Fig. 3. Chronic atopic dermatitis: lichenified plaques on the ankle.

disability-adjusted life years, which measure years of life lost due to premature mortality plus years lost due to disability or its consequences. All races are affected and people with "atopic tendency" often display a higher prevalence of hay fever, asthma, and food allergies.[20] Among populations, genetic studies show that AD affects diverse populations.[18]

Although AD most commonly affects children, all ages can be affected. In approximately 60% of cases, AD presents in the first year of life.[19,21,22] About 57% of children develop AD before age 6.[22]

WORLDWIDE/REGIONAL INCIDENCE AND MORTALITY RATES

There seems to be an association between higher socioeconomic status and AD prevalence and morbidity. Lifetime prevalence worldwide of AD is greater than 15%, especially in wealthy developed countries.[18,23]

The prevalence of AD globally varies around the world. According to the latest available data, AD continues to increase in prevalence in young children, aged 6 to 7 years and 13 to 14 years, in low-income countries. Some of the countries in which this trend is noted are Latin America or in Southeast Asia.[24]

Studies show that AD is a prevalent problem all around the world, among infants, children, young adults, and adults. The global prevalence of AD is highest in younger

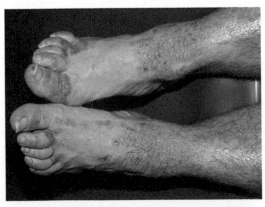

Fig. 4. Atopic dermatitis: thickened lichenified plaques on the ankles.

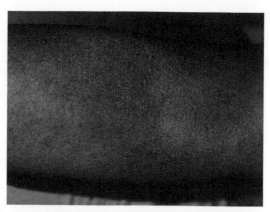

Fig. 5. Atopic dermatitis: lichenified plaques and hyperpigmentation of eczematous patch.

children compared with older children, adolescents, and adults. The significant predictors of AD were age, weather, food, race, ethnicity, place of birth, sex, current working status, and family history of atopy and maternal age.[25]

DISCUSSION
Goals of Treatment

The primary goals of treatment of AD are to reduce skin inflammation and pruritus, restore skin barrier function, and improve quality of life.[26] As previously discussed, treatments can be classified into the categories of moisturizing and basic skin care, topical therapies, phototherapy, and systemic therapies.[26–28] Reduction of itching and burning, as well as complete clearing of all skin changes, are the most important treatment goals for patients.[29]

Approach

The optimal management of AD requires a multipronged approach that involves the elimination of exacerbating factors, restoration of the skin barrier function and hydration of the skin, patient education, and pharmacologic treatment of skin inflammation.

AD is a chronic disease that can first present in childhood and persist across a lifetime with exacerbations. The general approach toward the treatment of AD is to reduce symptoms of inflammation and pruritis, prevent exacerbations, and limit the side effects of therapies to improve the overall quality of life.[26,29] The primary approach includes the avoidance of potential triggers and skin care with emollients to limit water loss, restore the epidermal barrier, and spare the use of steroids in exacerbations. Topical therapies include the use of TCS and calcineurin inhibitors.[28] Topic calcineurin inhibitors are second-line and are useful in patients who have not responded to TCS, in sensitive areas (eg, face, anogenital, skin folds), sites with steroid-associated atrophy, and long-term uninterrupted TCS use.[28] Phototherapy is recommended in children and adults for both acute and chronic AD not responding to topical therapies.[30] Systemic immunomodulatory agents are indicated in adult and pediatric patients in whom optimized topical regimens using emollients, topical anti-inflammatory therapies, adjunctive methods, and/or phototherapy do not provide adequate disease control.[30]

Evaluation

Dermoscopy of AD often shows focal white scales, yellow serous crust, and dotted vessels distributed in clusters or randomly with associated dilated capillaries in

Table 2
Frequently used topical corticosteroids for atopic dermatitis treatment

Classification	Topical Corticosteroid
Class 1 Very High Potency	• Augmented betamethasone dipropionate 0.05% (ointment, gel) • Augmented diflorasone diacetate 0.05% (ointment) • Clobetasol propionate 0.05% (ointment, gel, cream, lotion, foam, solution, spray, shampoo) • Desoximetasone 0.25% (spray) • Fluocinonide 0.1% (cream) • Flurandrenolide 4 µg/cm² (tape) • Halobetasol propionate 0.05% (ointment, cream)
Class 2	• Amcinonide 0.1% (ointment) • Augmented diflorasone diacetate 0.05% (cream) • Augmented betamethasone dipropionate 0.5% (cream, lotion) • Betamethasone dipropionate 0.05% (ointment) • Desoximetasone 0.05% (gel) • Desoximetasone 0.25% (ointment, cream) • Diflorasone diacetate 0.05% (ointment) • Fluocinonide 0.05% (ointment, gel, cream, lotion, solution) • Halcinonide 0.1% (ointment cream) • Mometasone fluroate 0.1% (ointment) • Triamcinolone acetonide 0.5% (ointment)
Class 3	• Amcinonide 0.1% (cream, lotion) • Betamethasone dipropionate 0.05% (cream, lotion) • Betamethasone valerate 0.1% (ointment) • Betamethasone valerate 0.12% (foam) • Diflorasone diacetate 0.05% (cream) • Fluticasone propionate 0.005% (ointment) • Triamcinolone acetonide 0.1% (ointment) • Triamcinolone acetonide 0.5% (cream)
Class 4	• Betamethasone valerate 0.12% (foam) • Desoximetasone 0.05% (cream) • Fluocinolone acetonide 0.025% (ointment) • Flurandrenolide 0.05% (ointment) • Hydrocortisone valerate 0.2% (ointment) • Mometasone furoate 0.1% (cream, lotion) • Triamcinolone acetonide 0.1% (ointment, cream) • Triamcinolone acetonide 0.2% (spray)
Class 5	• Betamethasone dipropionate 0.05% (lotion) • Betamethasone valerate 0.1% (cream, lotion) • Clocortolone pivalate 0.1% (cream) • Fluocinolone acetonide 0.025% (cream) • Fluocinolone acetonide 0.01% (oil, shampoo) • Fluticasone propionate 0.05% (cream, lotion) • Flurandrenolide 0.05% (cream) • Hydrocortisone butyrate 0.1% (ointment, cream, lotion, solution) • Hydrocortisone probutate 0.1% (cream) • Hydrocortisone valerate 0.2% (cream) • Prednicarbate 0.1% (ointment, cream) • Triamcinolone acetonide 0.025% (ointment) • Triamcinolone acetonide 0.01% (lotion)

(continued on next page)

Table 2 (continued)	
Classification	**Topical Corticosteroid**
Class 6	• Alclometasone dipropionate 0.05% (ointment, cream) • Betamethasone valerate 0.05% (lotion) • Desonide 0.05% (ointment, gel, cream, lotion, foam) • Fluocinolone acetonide 0.01% (cream, solution) • Triamcinolone acetonide 0.025% (cream, lotion)
Class 7 Lowest Potency	• Dexamethasone sodium phosphate 0.1% (cream) • Hydrocortisone 0.5%–2.5% (ointment, gel, cream, lotion, foam) • Methylprednisolone acetate 0.25% (cream)

Adapted from Eichenfield LF, Tom WL, Berger TG, Krol A, Paller AS, Schwarzenberger K, Bergman JN, Chamlin SL, Cohen DE, Cooper KD, Cordoro KM, Davis DM, Feldman SR, Hanifin JM, Margolis DJ, Silverman RA, Simpson EL, Williams HC, Elmets CA, Block J, Harrod CG, Smith Begolka W, Sidbury R. Guidelines of care for the management of atopic dermatitis: section 2. Management and treatment of atopic dermatitis with topical therapies. J Am Acad Dermatol. 2014 Jul;71(1):116 to 32.

irregularly elongated dermal papillae. In cases where intense itching occurs, hemorrhages are also seen.[31] The diagnosis is primarily made through history and physical examination findings; however, skin biopsy may be useful in cases where there is uncertainty.

Current Clinical Guidelines

Guidelines from the American Academy of Dermatology note that topical agents form the foundation of therapy for AD.[27,28,30] These include frequent use of topical moisturizers and effective bathing practices (duration and frequency are nonstandardized but it is recommended to apply moisturizers soon after bathing and limit the use of non-soap cleansers). TCS are the mainstay of topical anti-inflammatory treatment. It is generally recommended to apply twice daily, applying every day during flares, and once or twice weekly afterward to prevent recurrence. Topical calcineurin inhibitors include tacrolimus and pimecrolimus, second-line agents that have been approved for moderate-to-severe and mild-to-moderate AD, respectively. These do not carry the risk of skin atrophy that topical steroids do, making them potentially advantageous options in sensitive areas but commonly cause localized stinging/burning. Topical antimicrobials/antiseptics have generally not been shown to be effective, with the exception that diluted bleach baths seem to improve clinical outcomes in those with moderate-to-severe AD who have frequent bacterial skin infections.[28]

Phototherapy is a second-line treatment that has also been shown to be effective for AD. Many types of light and protocols for therapy can be used, with limited comparison trials available. It can be used on either an intermittent or continuous basis, as monotherapy or in combination with emollients and topical steroids (it is recommended to avoid combining it with topical calcineurin inhibitors). Side effects are low but it can cause erythema, burning, itching, and actinic damage.[30]

Further Treatment Options

Exciting new medications are now approved for moderate-to-severe AD. Dupilumab (Dupixent) is now FDA approved for patients with AD aged 6 months and older. It is an injection given 2 weeks apart and has a good safety profile with conjunctivitis being the most common side effect. In two phase 3 trials, the human monoclonal antibody against interleukin-4 receptor alpha dupilumab was shown to improve pruritus and

Table 3 Therapeutic approaches		
Mild AD	**Moderate AD**	**Severe AD**
Intermittent, short-term use of class 6 or 7 topical steroids (see Table) ± topical calcineurin inhibitors	Intermittent, short-term use of class 3–4 topical steroids (see Table) ± topical calcineurin inhibitors	Class 2 topical steroids for flares (see Table); class 3–5 topical steroids ± tacrolimus ointment for maintenance
Bathing and barrier repair with emollients	Oral antihistamines	Oral antihistamines
Avoidance of irritant and allergic triggers	Bathing and barrier repair	Bathing and barrier repair
Treat superinfection	Avoidance of irritant and allergic triggers	Avoidance of irritant and allergic triggers
	Treat superinfection	Treat superinfection
		Consider systemic anti-inflammatory agents, ultraviolet light therapy, biologics

Adapted from Paller A, Mancini AJ. Chapter 3 – Eczematous Eruptions in Childhood. Hurwitz Clinical Pediatric Dermatology: A Textbook of Skin Disorders of Childhood and Adolescence. 5th edition. Elsevier; 2015: 38-72e7.

increase the likelihood of achieving decreased scores on the Investigator's Global Assessment. In patients 18 years of age and older, dupilumab is administered 300 mg every other week via subcutaneous injection (after a 600 mg loading dose).[32] Dosing for the pediatric population is weight-based. Although crisaborole and dupilumab are FDA approved, their cost (ranging from US$700–3000 per month) make them impractical for many patients.[1]

JAK inhibitors such as upadacitinib and abrocitinib have been used with great success in moderate-to-severe AD.[33,34] Abrocitinib is an oral medication taken at doses of 100 or 200 mg once per day.[33] Side effect includes immunosuppression and potentially increased risk of upper respiratory tract infection, blood clots, and elevated liver enzymes. There are many other targeted treatments such as IL-13 and IL-31 inhibitors that are undergoing clinical trials.

An ointment of crisaborole (a phosphodiesterase 4 inhibitor) was found to be effective at reducing itching faster than vehicle alone; however, it is expensive and burning is a common complaint.[35]

Therapeutic Options

(Tables 2 and 3)

SUMMARY

AD is an extremely common skin condition that significantly decreases quality of life for both the patient and their caregivers. It is important for the primary care provider to be knowledgeable on the condition and its diagnosis and management/treatment options that are available.

Emollients such as creams and ointments are extremely important for the maintenance of patients with AD. For AD flares, TCS are considered first-line treatment. In moderate and severe AD, topical calcineurin inhibitors can be used in combination with topical steroids as a steroid-sparing therapy or for areas with thin skin such as the face and intertriginous areas. Second-line treatment of moderate and severe AD that can be used is Ultraviolet light B (UVB) phototherapy. For severe AD, dupilumab is an established and effective treatment option, and Janus kinase (JAK) inhibitors are also approved and effective for severe AD. Immunosuppressants such as metho-trexate, azathioprine, mycophenolate mofetil, and cyclosporine can be used for AD but they all have their own side effect profile.

Routine evaluation of AD should not include blood tests or skin prick tests. Although secondary infection is the most common complication of AD, without evidence for clinical infection in patients with AD, oral antibiotics should not be used. Lichenifica-tion and postinflammatory scarring can be seen in chronic AD. Long-term treatment of AD should not include systemic corticosteroids.

Noncompliance to treatment regimens effect treatment outcomes and patients. Every effort should be made to assess the multifactorial issues that contribute to noncompliance for a patient including cost, patient bias, complex regimens, infre-quent follow-up, and lack of knowledge. Frequent follow-ups, patient education, and AD action plans can help improve patient outcomes through adherence.[1] Because this is a common and chronic condition, primary care physicians should be aware of its diagnosis and treatment and be able to set realistic expectations for these patients.

CLINICS CARE POINTS

- The diagnosis of AD is primarily based on history and physical examination findings. SORT C
- Skincare, emollients, and avoidance of triggers are recommended in all patients for chronic treatment. SORT A
- TCS are first-line treatments during AD exacerbations. SORT A
- Topic calcineurin inhibitors are useful in patients who have not responded to TCS, and for maintenance therapy in sensitive areas (eg, face, anogenital, skin folds), sites with steroid-associated atrophy, and long-term uninterrupted TCS use. SORT A
- Monoclonal antibody treatments are effective in patients with moderate-to-severe AD not responsive to topical therapies. SORT A

DISCLOSURE

The authors have nothing to disclose.

ACKNOWLEDGMENTS

The authors would like to thank the Penn State Health Milton S. Hershey Medical Cen-ter Department of Dermatology for the contribution of the photographs for this article.

REFERENCES

1. Frazier W, Bhardwaj N. Atopic Dermatitis: Diagnosis and Treatment. Am Fam Physician 2020;101(10):590–8.
2. Brunner PM, Silverberg JI, Guttman-Yassky E, et al. Increasing Comorbidities Suggest that Atopic Dermatitis Is a Systemic Disorder. J Invest Dermatol 2017; 137(1):18–25.
3. Yaghmaie P, Koudelka CW, Simpson EL. Mental Health Comorbidity in Atopic Dermatitis. J Allergy Clin Immunol 2013;131(2):428.
4. Avena-Woods C. Overview of atopic dermatitis. Am J Manag Care 2017;23(8 Suppl):S115–23.

5. Elias PM, Hatano Y, Williams ML. Basis for the barrier abnormality in atopic dermatitis: Outside-inside-outside pathogenic mechanisms. J Allergy Clin Immunol 2008;121(6):1337.

6. Bieber T. Atopic dermatitis. N Engl J Med 2008;358(14):1483–94.

7. Morar N, Cookson WOCM, Harper JI, et al. Filaggrin Mutations in Children with Severe Atopic Dermatitis. J Invest Dermatol 2007;127(7):1667–72.

8. Vickery BP. Skin barrier function in atopic dermatitis. Curr Opin Pediatr 2007; 19(1):89–93.

9. Davari DR, Nieman EL, McShane DB, et al. Current Perspectives on the Management of Infantile Atopic Dermatitis. J Asthma Allergy 2020;13:563.

10. Lyons JJ, Milner JD, Stone KD. Atopic dermatitis in children: clinical features, pathophysiology, and treatment. Immunol Allergy Clin N Am 2015;35(1):161–83.

11. Williams HC, Jburney PG, Hay RJ, et al. The U.K. Working Party's Diagnostic Criteria for Atopic Dermatitis. I. Derivation of a minimum set of discriminators for atopic dermatitis. Br J Dermatol 1994;131(3):383–96.

12. Vakharia PP, Chopra R, Silverberg JI. Systematic Review of Diagnostic Criteria Used in Atopic Dermatitis Randomized Controlled Trials. Am J Clin Dermatol 2018;19(1):15–22.

13. Hanifln JM. Diagnostic features of atopic dermatitis. Acta Derm Venereol 1980; 92:44–7.

14. Du Toit G, Roberts G, Sayre PH, et al, LEAP Study Team. Randomized trial of peanut consumption in infants at risk for peanut allergy. N Engl J Med 2015;372(9): 803–13. Erratum in: N Engl J Med. 2016 Jul 28;375(4):398.

15. Togias A, Cooper SF, Acebal ML, et al. Addendum guidelines for the prevention of peanut allergy in the United States: Report of the National Institute of Allergy and Infectious Diseases–sponsored expert panel. World Allergy Organ J 2017; 10(1):1.

16. Kristal L, Klein PA. Atopic dermatitis in infants and children. An update. Pediatr Clin North Am 2000;47(4):877–95.

17. Langan SM, Irvine AD, Weidinger S. Atopic dermatitis. Lancet 2020;396(10247): 345–60.

18. Asher MI, Montefort S, Björkstén B, et al. Worldwide time trends in the prevalence of symptoms of asthma, allergic rhinoconjunctivitis, and eczema in childhood: ISAAC Phases One and Three repeat multicountry cross-sectional surveys. Lancet 2006;368(9537):733–43.

19. Weidinger S, Novak N. Atopic dermatitis. Lancet 2016;387(10023):1109–22.

20. Silverberg JI, Hanifin JM. Adult eczema prevalence and associations with asthma and other health and demographic factors: a US population-based study. J Allergy Clin Immunol 2013;132(5):1132–8.

21. Illi S, von Mutius E, Lau S, et al. The natural course of atopic dermatitis from birth to age 7 years and the association with asthma. J Allergy Clin Immunol 2004; 113(5):925–31.

22. Garmhausen D, Hagemann T, Bieber T, et al. Characterization of different courses of atopic dermatitis in adolescent and adult patients. Allergy 2013;68(4):498–506.

23. Kaufman BP, Guttman-Yassky E, Alexis AF. Atopic dermatitis in diverse racial and ethnic groups-Variations in epidemiology, genetics, clinical presentation and treatment. Exp Dermatol 2018;27(4):340–57.

24. Nutten S. Atopic dermatitis: global epidemiology and risk factors. Ann Nutr Metab 2015;66(Suppl 1):8–16.

25. Hadi HA, Tarmizi AI, Khalid KA, et al. The Epidemiology and Global Burden of Atopic Dermatitis: A Narrative Review. Life 2021;11(9). https://doi.org/10.3390/LIFE11090936.
26. Dhadwal G, Albrecht L, Gniadecki R, et al. Approach to the assessment and management of adult patients with atopic dermatitis: A consensus document. Section IV: Treatment options for the management of atopic dermatitis. J Cutan Med Surg 2018;22:21S–9S.
27. Sidbury R, Tom WL, Bergman JN, et al. Guidelines of care for the management of atopic dermatitis: Section 4. Prevention of disease flares and use of adjunctive therapies and approaches. J Am Acad Dermatol 2014;71(6):1218–33.
28. Eichenfield LF, Tom WL, Berger TG, et al. Guidelines of care for the management of atopic dermatitis: section 2. Management and treatment of atopic dermatitis with topical therapies. J Am Acad Dermatol 2014;71(1):116–32.
29. Schmitt J, Csötönyi F, Bauer A, et al. Determinants of treatment goals and satisfaction of patients with atopic eczema. J Dtsch Dermatol Ges 2008;6(6):458–65.
30. Sidbury R, Davis DM, Cohen DE, et al. Guidelines of care for the management of atopic dermatitis: section 3. Management and treatment with phototherapy and systemic agents. J Am Acad Dermatol 2014;71(2):327–49.
31. Errichetti E. Dermoscopy of Inflammatory Dermatoses (Inflammoscopy): An Up-to-Date Overview. Dermatol Pract Concept 2019;9(3):169–80.
32. EL S, B A, M A. Two Phase 3 Trials of Dupilumab versus Placebo in Atopic Dermatitis. N Engl J Med 2017;376(11):1090–1.
33. Bieber T, Simpson EL, Silverberg JI, et al. Abrocitinib versus Placebo or Dupilumab for Atopic Dermatitis. N Engl J Med 2021;384(12):1101–12.
34. Guttman-Yassky E, Thaçi D, Pangan AL, et al. Upadacitinib in adults with moderate to severe atopic dermatitis: 16-week results from a randomized, placebo-controlled trial. J Allergy Clin Immunol 2020;145(3):877–84.
35. Paller AS, Tom WL, Lebwohl MG, et al. Efficacy and safety of crisaborole ointment, a novel, nonsteroidal phosphodiesterase 4 (PDE4) inhibitor for the topical treatment of atopic dermatitis (AD) in children and adults. J Am Acad Dermatol 2016;75(3):494–503, e6.

Food Allergy

Chelsea Elizabeth Mendonca, MD[a],*, Doerthe A. Andreae, MD, PhD[b]

KEYWORDS

- Food allergy • Anaphylaxis • IgE mediated • Skin prick test
- Epinephrine autoinjectors

KEY POINTS

- Food allergies are becoming increasingly more common in the United States.
- Although diagnostic testing can aid in diagnosis, a thorough clinical history is the most important step in diagnosis, as widespread testing can lead to false positives.
- There are no current cures for food allergy, and the mainstay of treatment involves avoidance of allergenic foods.
- There are many ongoing studies for advancements in diagnosis and treatments of food allergy to help improve quality of life.
- Food allergies have a large impact on the quality of life for not only patients but also their families.

INTRODUCTION

The National Institute of Allergy and Infectious Disease (NIAID) defines food allergy as "an adverse health effect arising from a specific immune response that occurs reproducibly on exposure to a given food." Food allergy affects many around the world, and the prevalence has been increasing.[1,2] The most detrimental manifestation of food allergy is anaphylaxis, which leads to the death of 150 to 200 people annually in the United States.[3,4] The diagnosis of food allergy can be difficult because available testing does not always correlate with clinical significance. Although there are no current treatments to cure food allergies, research is ongoing for new interventions to help improve the quality of life for these patients.

EPIDEMIOLOGY

Food allergies are becoming more common and affect up to 10% of the population in the United States.[1,2] The precise prevalence of food allergies is difficult to determine, as it would require analyses done with confirmatory oral food challenges, which is

[a] Department of Family and Community Medicine, Baylor College of Medicine, 1100 West 34th Street, Houston, TX 77018, USA; [b] Division of Allergy and Immunology, Department of Dermatology, University of Utah, 30 North 1900 East, 4A330, Salt Lake City, UT 84132, USA
* Corresponding author.
E-mail address: ChelseaMendoncaMD@gmail.com

Prim Care Clin Office Pract 50 (2023) 205–220
https://doi.org/10.1016/j.pop.2023.01.002
0095-4543/23/© 2023 Elsevier Inc. All rights reserved.

primarycare.theclinics.com

rarely done in the United States because of lack of feasibility and ethical issues.[5] Other objective methods do not always correlate with clinical significance. Because of the lack of objective data, many studies use self-reported food allergy rates, which are substantially higher than those confirmed by objective methods.[1,6] There have been no prevalence studies conducted in the United States using the gold standard for food allergy diagnosis, the oral food challenge.[5] There has also been an increase in hospitalizations in recent years for food-induced anaphylaxis.[5,7–9] Geographic variations in prevalence are likely due to diet exposure effects, differences according to age, race, ethnicity, and other factors.[1,10–12] The World Allergy Organization found that the rates for food allergy are lowest in Thailand and Iceland, whereas highest in Canada, Australia, and Finland.

PATHOPHYSIOLOGY

Food allergies can be divided into immunoglobulin E (IgE)-mediated and non–IgE-mediated food allergies. It is important to note that food allergies are different from food intolerances, which are not discussed in this article.

In normal food tolerance, food antigens cross the mucosal barrier and are processed by dendritic cells in a nonactivated state that induces the suppression of cytokines by antigen-presenting cells; this results in differentiation of naïve T cells into regulatory T cells and suppression of food antigen–specific TH2 cells as well as increased IgA and IgG4 production with a decrease in IgE production by B cells. This process leads to a suppression of eosinophils, basophils, and mast cells.[1,13–17]

Sensitization is the state of having a detectable food-specific IgE level, which is a precursor to the development of clinical food allergy. There are many players in the development of sensitization.[13] IgE-mediated food allergies are a result of the loss of integrity of key immune components that maintain a state of tolerance to foreign proteins in healthy individuals. In affected individuals, commonly benign food antigens are recognized as pathogenic and produce clinical symptoms. Food-specific IgE binds to receptors on mast cells and basophils and releases preformed mediators into the circulation that play a role in the clinical findings.[1,13,18]

- Histamine has a rapid onset of action (usually within 5 minutes) and leads to vasodilation and increased vascular permeability, which leads to the increased heart rate, increased cardiac contraction, and increased glandular secretion.[13]
- Tryptase levels tend to peak at 60 to 90 minutes and has limited diffusion from an activated mast cell, so it leads to more localized symptoms such as angioedema.[13]
- Platelet-activating factor leads to bronchoconstriction, increased vascular permeability, chemotaxis, and degranulation of eosinophils and neutrophils. It is a potent mediator of anaphylaxis.[13]
- Prostaglandins PGD2 is produced by mast cells and leads to bronchoconstriction, peripheral vasodilation, and coronary and pulmonary artery vasoconstriction.[13]
- Leukotrienes have a slow onset of action and lead to smooth muscle contraction, mucous secretion, and an increase in vascular permeability.[13]

Non–IgE-mediated food allergies include disorders such as eosinophilic esophagitis, food protein–induced enterocolitis syndrome (FPIES), or food protein–induced proctocolitis.[1] The pathophysiology behind non–IgE-mediated food allergies is not completely understood. FPIES is characterized by delayed, profuse vomiting and can be misdiagnosed. It usually resolves spontaneously.[1] Eosinophilic esophagitis can present with dysphagia, which can lead patients to suspect that the food that led to the response is allergenic in nature, but a small number of foods account for most of the inflammation in patients with eosinophilic esophagitis.[1]

RISK FACTORS

Identifying the risk factors is an important part of the diagnostic workup for patients with food allergies. One of the strongest risk factors is a family history of atopy. One immediate family member with any allergic disease increases the risk of food allergy by 40% and up to 80% in patients with 2 immediate family members with any allergic disease[5,19]; 66.6% of children with food allergic siblings were found to be food sensitized, but only 13.6% were clinically reactive.[20,21] The genetic determinants of food allergy are still not fully understood.[5]

Other risk factors associated with food allergies include male sex, Asian and Black race, genetic factors such as familial associations, human leukocyte antigen, comorbid atopic dermatitis and asthma, and specific genes.[1,5,19,22–26] In attempts to reduce or prevent food allergies, research on potentially modifiable risk factors has investigated vitamin D insufficiency, dietary fat consumption, consumption of antioxidants, use of antacids, and obesity.[1] Timing of introduction of food allergens in infancy/early childhood has been found to be an important measure.

Environmental factors can also be associated with food allergy risk.[5,20] Children with siblings and pets in the home were found to be at lower risk of food allergies compared with those without siblings and pets. Children growing up in a rural environment with close contact to livestock have also been shown to have lower rates. Another interesting implication has been parental nativity. Children born in the United States or who immigrated in early childhood had higher odds of sensitization than foreign-born children. Children born to immigrant parents also had higher odds of sensitization.[5,27]

Studies determining the role of the gut microbial environments' association with food sensitization and allergies have found that certain microbiota such as Lactococcus and Citrobacter may be underrepresented in patients with food allergies.[28,29]

EVALUATION
Elements of the History

The most important single "test" for diagnosing food allergy is a thorough clinical history.[1] Understanding the clinical manifestations of IgE-mediated food allergies compared with non–IgE-mediated food allergies and food intolerances helps the clinician to determine which next steps are the most beneficial for each patient. For most patients, symptoms of IgE-mediated food allergies usually occur within minutes to 1 to 2 hours after exposure to the food.[28] The most common food allergens are milk, egg, peanut, tree nuts, wheat, soy, fish, and shellfish. A detailed history should be taken including factors pertaining to the most recent reaction but also regarding diet, past reactions, and family history. Important elements of the clinical history can be found in **Table 1**.

There is a strong association between atopic dermatitis and the development of food allergies especially in children with severe atopic dermatitis in the first 3 months of life.[13,30,31] Clinical and family history provides the necessary information to determine the necessity for testing and potentially further management.[13]

Signs and Symptoms

Food allergies often can affect multiple systems throughout the body. Reactions range from mild symptoms to severe anaphylaxis and even death if not treated quickly and

Table 1 Important elements of the clinical history	
Aspects	**Questions**
Most recent reaction	• What were the presenting symptoms? • How long did they last? • Which foods were ingested before the reactions? • Has the patient reacted to this food before and more than once? • What was the amount of food ingested? • How long after ingestion of the food did the symptoms occur? • Was the reaction to baked or uncooked food? • Has the food ever been eaten before without the occurrence of symptoms? • Were there any factors such as recent illness, activity, alcohol consumption, use of aspirin or NSAIDs?
Previous reactions	• Had the food been tolerated in the past in the absence of the aforementioned factors, specifically activity? • Has the patient ever developed symptoms after being exposed to another food? • Does the patient avoid any specific foods?
Atopic and other comorbidities	• What other atopic conditions does the patient have (eg, asthma, allergic rhinitis, atopic dermatitis, eosinophilic esophagitis) • Does the patient have any other medical problems?
Previous diagnostic tests	• Has the patient ever had food allergy testing, if yes, which ones and what were the results? • Has the patient received any immunotherapy for food allergies, either for peanut or as part of a study or off-label use?
Available treatments	• Does the patient carry an epinephrine autoinjector? • Does the patient and the family know how to use it? • Do they have a food allergy emergency plan? • Are they familiar with symptoms of food allergy and anaphylaxis and the required interventions?
Family history	• Do parents or siblings have food allergies? • Are any foods avoided in the patient's diet because of an allergy in a family member?

Abbreviation: NSAIDs, nonsteroidal antiinflammatory drugs.

appropriately. Many patients associate any reaction to food as a food allergy, and differentiating immune-mediated food allergies from non–immune-mediated food allergies helps to determine further testing and management.

Cutaneous symptoms are the most common presenting symptoms for food allergies. The severity of the cutaneous symptoms is determined by the percentage of skin involved in the reaction.[13,32] Manifestations include erythematous rashes, pruritus, urticaria, and angioedema. Mild symptoms include occasional scratching or persistent pruritus. Hives may or may not be present. Hives usually occur immediately after ingestion of the culprit food and can last for hours without treatment.[13] Angioedema usually presents with swelling of the eyelid, face, and/or lip and can cause significant discomfort.[13] Rashes such as erythematous macular rash and eczematous rashes are also symptoms of IgE-mediated food allergies, but non–IgE-mediated immune mechanisms also play a role.[13]

Ocular involvement can also be seen in patients presenting with food allergies. Lacrimation, eye redness, and itching are common mild presentations. Severe ocular manifestations include significant periorbital swelling.[13,33]

Respiratory involvement is commonly present and can be an indication of more severe reactions. Nasal symptoms can range from occasional sniffing or rubbing of the nose to moderate to severe symptoms, such as persistent rhinorrhea, nasal congestion, or a complete blockage of the nasal passage.[13] Lower respiratory symptoms include expiratory wheezing, coughing, use of accessory muscles for breathing, and even severe asthma exacerbations.[13] Laryngeal symptoms include throat clearing, cough, throat tightness, or throat pain. More severe symptoms include hoarseness and dry, persistent cough. The most severe symptom is stridor with complete airway obstructions.[13]

The most severe manifestations of food allergies include symptoms of dizziness or weakness. Objective signs of cardiovascular or neurologic involvement include tachycardia, hypotension, changes in mental status, severe cardiovascular collapse, unconsciousness, or even death. It is rare that these symptoms are present without involvement of other organs such as respiratory or cutaneous manifestations.[13] Cardiovascular and neurologic symptoms are considered symptoms of severe food allergic reactions.[13]

Gastrointestinal symptoms can also be associated with food allergies but must be differentiated from food intolerances. Subjective symptoms include itching of the mouth or throat, nausea, or abdominal pain. Objective symptoms include vomiting and diarrhea. Symptoms are usually immediately present if associated with IgE-mediated food allergies and occur within minutes to no more than 4 hours.[13] Failure to thrive, bloody diarrhea, constipation, weight loss, long-term malabsorption, emesis, or diarrhea that occur more than 4 hours after food ingestion are typically associated with non–IgE-mediated food allergies.[13]

The most severe presentation of food allergies is anaphylaxis. Anaphylaxis is an IgE-mediated hypersensitivity reaction that involves multiple organ systems. It is rapid in onset and potentially fatal if interventions are delayed. Cardiovascular or neurologic symptoms are also more commonly present in association with anaphylaxis.

Exercise-induced anaphylaxis is present in about one-third of food allergic adults.[13] These patients can usually tolerate the allergenic food in the absence of exercise. The most common symptoms associated with exercise-induced anaphylaxis are pruritus, urticaria, angioedema, flushing, and shortness of breath.

Diagnostic Testing

Once the clinical history is obtained, diagnostic testing can be used to confirm the presence of food allergies and guide management. Many primary care physicians feel uncomfortable in interpreting laboratory tests when diagnosing food allergy.[1,34] It is important to choose diagnostic testing carefully, as ordering large panels of diagnostic tests can lead to false-positive results and unnecessary dietary eliminations that have many implications.[13]

The gold standard for diagnosing food allergies is the oral food challenge.[5] A negative test occurs when the patient does not develop any objective symptoms during the challenge but interpretation must be correlated with the patient's history.[5] Food challenges should only be carried out under the supervision of medical personnel who have experience in interpretation of symptoms and management of reactions. Oral food challenges often help improve quality of life even when resulting in an allergic reaction.[1,35–38] Failing the oral challenge can lead to increased comfort in recognizing and treating food allergic reactions. It is important to counsel families that a reaction from an oral food challenge does not result in increased sensitization to that food.[1,39–41]

The most used test is the skin prick/puncture tests (SPT).[28,42] SPTs are performed to determine culprit foods when a patient's history is suggestive of a possible food allergy. A 4- to 6-week waiting period after an anaphylaxis reaction should be given before skin testing is performed to ensure restoration of skin reactivity.[13] The wheal is measured 15 minutes after the prick was applied. The diameter of the wheal indicates the likelihood of clinical reactivity, not the severity of a potential allergic reaction. A positive skin test is defined as the mean diameter at least 3 mm larger than the negative control.[13,42] Some pitfalls to skin testing include low specificity, low positive predictive value, and lack of standardization of reagents and methods. Although SPTs detect the presence of food allergen–specific IgE, patients can have IgE in the absence of clinical symptoms. False negatives can be seen with skin testing. If the history is significant, diagnosis should be confirmed using other testing.[28] The use of SPT alone in the clinical setting is not diagnostic and can result in overdiagnosis.[13,28,43]

IgE testing measures the allergen-specific IgE antibody levels in the patient's blood. The presence of IgE antibodies indicates allergic sensitization and does not necessarily mean clinical reactivity. IgE levels may correlate directly with the probability of a clinical reaction, so high levels may suggest ingestion of the food in question will lead to an allergic reaction.[28,44] Results tend to vary between different laboratories so they are not comparable, and predictive values from one assay cannot be applied to other test methods.[28,45] The sensitivity of this testing is greater than 90%; however, specificity is less than 50% due to possible cross-reactivity between related proteins.[13]

New testing is being developed to assist with the diagnosis of food allergies. Some tests currently being studied include the following:

- *Molecular or component-resolved diagnostics (CRD)* tests have been used to evaluate reactions to specific proteins. IgE binding to specific proteins might provide more specific diagnostic information than tests that report IgE binding to extracts compromised of mixtures of proteins.[1] Foods are composed of numerous proteins, and individuals with a food allergy may have a response of varying degrees to any of the proteins. Proteins easily destroyed by heating or digestion may be less likely to cause significant reactions compared with those that are more stable. CRD for specific food allergens such as peanut and hazelnut is being used in clinical practice to help distinguish between true food allergy and pollen-food allergy syndrome.

In children at high risk of food allergies, it is not recommended to obtain routine testing before introducing highly allergenic foods, as widespread testing has poor predictive value.[28,46] There are some cases when food allergy evaluation can be helpful before introduction of foods such as in children who have a sibling with a food allergy or patients who have another coexisting food allergy or specific comorbid condition.[28,47] The greatest source of misdiagnosis of food allergies comes from the lack of understanding that a positive test result does not conclusively diagnose food allergy and that testing might have been performed for food allergens the patient had been consuming without reaction.[1]

CROSS-REACTIVITY

Cross-reactivity between food and pollen can result in observation of positive test results that might not have clinical implications that can affect interpretation. Legumes, for example, have a high level of homologous proteins compared with other beans and yet individual patients may only react to distinct types.[1] Allergies to cockroach or dust mites may result in positive results to crustacean shellfish.[1]

Pollen-food allergy syndrome is an IgE-mediated allergic reaction against fruits and plants that has been linked to sensitization to inhaled plant allergens.[48] Symptoms most commonly affect the oral mucosa, but the gastrointestinal, respiratory, and cardiovascular system can also be involved. Symptoms develop within 5 to 10 minutes following raw food intake; however, patients are able to tolerate cooked or processed versions of that plant food.[48] The diagnosis should be considered in patients who suffer from a pollen allergy. Sensitization to the pollen occurs, and later in life, food allergies are noted due to cross-reactivities. See **Table 2** for cross-reactivity patterns.

MANAGEMENT/TREATMENT

Although there are not definitive cures for food allergies, symptoms can be treated, reactions avoided, and, in some cases, sustained nonresponsiveness can be achieved. Antihistamines are commonly used for mild reactions to food, and patients often feel comfortable self-administering these.

Anaphylaxis

For all patients with food allergies, the most important step is identifying anaphylaxis, which can be life-threatening. Teaching patients about recognizing anaphylaxis and treatment options outside of the hospital have been shown to decrease hospitalizations. The first-line therapy for anaphylaxis is intramuscular (IM) epinephrine. Epinephrine works by vasoconstricting blood vessels to maintain blood pressure, bronchodilation of the airway to improve respirations, and decreases edema that can lead to airway collapse. In the clinical setting the most appropriate dose is 0.01 to 0.03 mg/kg, with a maximum dose of 0.5 mg injected intramuscularly into the thigh.

All patients with food allergy should be prescribed an epinephrine autoinjector to use in the event of accidental exposure.[13] Autoinjectors for patients are available in the 0.1 mg, 0.15 mg, and 0.3 mg doses. For those patients less than 30 kg, the 0.15 mg dose is recommended and those greater than 30 kg should be prescribed the 0.3 mg dose.[13,49] The infant dose of 0.1 mg can be used for infants and toddlers up to 10 kg. Studies have shown that epinephrine is underused during anaphylaxis by patients.[1,45] The reluctance if often related to fear of needles and side effects of the medication.[1,50] Improved use of epinephrine autoinjectors is seen when adolescents

Table 2 Foods associated with tree pollens	
Birch	Apple, peach, apricot, cherry, plum, pear, almond hazelnut, carrot, celery, parsley, caraway, fennel, coriander, aniseed, soybean, peanut, jackfruit
Plane	Hazelnut, peach, apricot, plum, apple, kiwi, peanut, corn, chickpea, lettuce, green beans
Japanese cedar	Tomato
Cypress pollen	Peach, citrus fruit
Ragweed	Cantaloupe, honeydew, watermelon, zucchini, cucumber, bananas
Mugwort	Carrot, celery, parsley, caraway, fennel, coriander, aniseed, bell pepper, black pepper, garlic, onion, mango, paprika, peach, lychee, grape, sunflower seeds
Grass pollen	Melons, white potato, tomato, orange, swiss chard, peanut, kiwi

are able to practice self-injection in the office to address issues such as needle phobia.[1,51] Patients should also be counseled that self-injectable epinephrine is safe and efficacious and patients should be comfortable using it liberally. Use of prehospital epinephrine has been associated with less likelihood of hospitalization and poor outcomes.[1,52]

Acute management of patients with anaphylaxis also consists of vital sign monitoring, supplemental oxygen, fluid resuscitation, and cardiopulmonary resuscitation.[13,49] H1-antihistamines are the next treatment that should be used for anaphylactic symptoms. They can relieve symptoms as a single agent or in addition with H2-antihistamines. By blocking H1 and H2 receptors, blood pressure and heart rate can be maintained by increased vascular integrity.[13,53] It is very important to educate patients not to delay the use of epinephrine. Although glucocorticoids are commonly used in the emergency, there is a lack of evidence for clear benefit.[13] See **Table 3** for anaphylaxis treatment.

Avoidance

The most effective long-term management strategy is strict food allergen avoidance. For most patients, the reason for a subsequent reaction following a confirmed diagnosis is failure to avoid the known allergen. Patients should be counseled, preferably by a registered dietitian, about strategies and vigilance required to avoid specific food allergens and appropriate substitutes.[13] Part of the avoidance strategy includes learning to read food labels. Teenagers and young adults are considered high risk for fatal reactions because of risk-taking behavior and lack of prompt treatment.[1,54] Two methods that have been shown to improve adhere include engaging in a support group and having an anaphylaxis management plan with their physician.[1,55]

In patients eliminating foods from the diet, it is important to monitor for nutritional deficiencies especially if multiple foods are omitted.[28,56] In those who do not receive

Table 3
Management of anaphylaxis

First-Line Treatment	Second-Line Treatment	Third-Line Treatment
Epinephrine (epi) autoinjector, IM in the anterolateral thigh, or IM epi of a 1:1000 solution	Bronchodilator, eg, albuterol as MDI or nebulized solution	H1-antihistamine, first or second generation, PO or IV, liquid preferred over tablets
Autoinjector dosing: 1.1 mg for <10 kg 0.15 mg for 10–30 kg 0.3 mg for >30 kg and adult	Albuterol MDI dosing: 4–8 puffs children 8 puffs adolescent and adult	For example, diphenhydramine 1–2 mg/kg with max dose of 50 mg
Epi 1:1000 solution dosing: 0.01 mg/kg per dose: maximum dose, 0.5 mg per dose	Nebulized solution dosing: 1.5 mL children 3 mL adolescent and adult	For example, cetirizine 2.5 mg infants 5 mg children 10 mg adolescent and adult
Injection can be repeated after 5–20 min	Every 20 min or continuously	—
• Supplemental oxygen as needed • Recumbent position with elevated legs • IV fluids for hypotension, orthostasis, or poor response to epi		

Abbreviation: MDI, metered-dose inhaler.

nutritional counseling, there is an increased risk of inadequate intake specifically seen with calcium and vitamin D and increased risk for malnutrition and reduced height.[1,57]

Oral Immunotherapy

Oral immunotherapy (OIT) is an emerging treatment of food allergy that involves introducing the allergen in an oral vehicle such as in milk or powder form. Doses are increased slowly over 2- to 4-week intervals in order to build tolerance to the food. Patients would ideally be able to ingest the food without anaphylaxis symptoms.[13] In a randomized controlled trial published in the Lancet 2014, desensitization was noted to be higher in the OIT group compared with the control group, and quality-of-life scores improved, showing efficacy of OIT.[13,58]

Emerging Treatments

There are many emerging treatments that are being evaluated currently for food allergies to achieve sustained unresponsiveness:

Epicutaneous immunotherapy involves placing a patch with food allergen on the skin in an attempt to promote systemic tolerance, as the food allergen is absorbed through the skin. Randomized controlled trials have shown efficacy to induce systemic tolerance to peanuts after 12 months of therapy. This method is currently under evaluation.[13,59]

Sublingual immunotherapy (SLIT) involves placing food proteins under the tongue in increasing doses. It is currently being compared with oral immunotherapy. OIT has shown a significantly greater increase in food challenge tolerance thresholds, but SLIT has been associated with fewer adverse reactions.[13,60]

Omalizumab is an anti-IgE antibody that is being studied as monotherapy to alter reactivity. Studies thus far have shown an increase in thresholds, but more studies are needed to evaluate the benefits.[1,61]

Developing Tolerance

Overtime, some patients may develop a tolerance to foods that were previously allergy inducing. Some factors that have been predictive for developing tolerance include the severity of the symptoms on ingestion, the skin prick test size, the age of diagnosis, comorbid allergic disease and severity, food-specific IgE levels, and the rate of change of food-specific IgE levels or skin prick test sizes over time since diagnosis.[5] In order to determine whether tolerance has developed, oral food challenges are usually necessary for confirmation. IgE-based methods are often imprecise and cannot be used for clinical significance.[5]

Vaccinations in Patients with Egg Allergy

Primary care physicians are at the forefront of vaccination, and understanding contraindications to vaccines is an important part of preventative medicine. There are many misconceptions regarding the safety of vaccines in children with food allergies.

Influenza vaccine, both the inactivated influenza vaccine and the live-attenuated influenza vaccine, are safe for people living with egg allergies. It is not necessary to ask about food allergy before the administration of influenza vaccine, and the severity of the allergy does not affect one's ability to receive the vaccine.[28,62,63]

MMR and MMR-V can both be safely administered to children with egg allergies of any severity.[28]

Yellow fever vaccine is contraindicated in patients with egg allergies. For those who need the vaccine, allergy evaluation and testing can be done with the vaccine itself to determine if the patient can receive it.[28,64]

Rabies vaccine has 3 different types. The purified chick embryo cell culture vaccine is contraindicated in patients who are allergic to eggs. It can be safely administered if an allergy evaluation and testing is done with the vaccine itself.[28,64] It is recommended to use the human diploid cell vaccine or purified vero cell vaccine for rabies prophylaxis.

PREVENTION

As the prevalence of food allergy increases, there has been an important emphasis placed on determining ways to prevent the development of food allergies. One of the biggest factors that has been examined is the proper timing of food introduction to infants to help minimize food allergies. The American Academy of Allergy, Asthma, and Immunology generally recommends introducing of complementary foods between the ages of 4 and 6 months, with highly allergenic foods introduced in small quantities at home, once other foods are tolerated. It is important to note that some young infants may demonstrate clinical allergy to foods on their first exposure. The optimal time to introduce allergenic foods is not known.

The American Academy of Pediatrics does not recommend delaying introduction of highly allergenic complimentary foods as a tactic to prevent development of food allergies.[5] Diversifying food exposure of infants may be associated with a protective effect on food sensitization and clinical food allergy.[5,65] Breastfeeding has not been conclusively shown to have a protective role in preventing allergic disease, but exclusive breastfeeding is recommended for all infants until age 4 to 6 months.

The Learning Early About Peanut (LEAP) trial has been influential in discussing the introduction of allergenic foods to children at risk for developing food allergies. In the trial, infants ages 4 to 11 months at high risk for peanut allergies but with SPT testing of wheal size 4 mm or less were randomized to either consume peanuts or avoid peanut allergens until 5 years of age.[20,26,66] The results of this study provided the basis for the NIAID expert panel to evaluate for introduction of peanuts early to those at risk for development of peanut allergy; this is aligned with prior guidelines that recommended allergenic foods be introduced without any particular delay.[1,67,68] There are no specific current recommendations to purposely feed egg early or avoid eggs in the infant diet.[20,67,68] The data available on introduction of milk only suggests delayed introduction to be associated with increased risk of development of allergy.[20,69]

Other interventions have been studied and discussed in the literature. The Australian HealthNuts study found that infants with vitamin D deficiency may be at an increased risk for peanut and egg allergy. There are conflicting studies on the findings though. Therefore, ensuring vitamin D sufficiency could be a simple intervention to help prevent the development of food allergies but more data are needed.[20,70] Improving the skin barrier early through moisturizing the skin can also reduce the risk of eczema and theoretically food allergy via skin sensitization.[20,71,72]

QUALITY OF LIFE

Quality of life is an important factor for primary care physicians to consider when counseling families on food allergies. Discussions with parents and children about how the food allergy affects day-to-day life can help physicians build rapport and determine interventions that can lead to a better quality of life. A greater number of food allergies has been associated with a lower quality of life.[3]

Challenges that arise with attending school can have a profound impact on a child's development. Schools can serve as exposure to potential food triggers, which leads up to 10% of parents of children with food allergies to homeschool their children.[3]

Some schools have implemented the use of "peanut-free tables" for those children with allergies, which has been shown to be associated with a lower incidence rate of food allergy–related incidents compared with schools with no food policy.[13,73] However, the use of "peanut-free tables" can lead to social isolation for children and worsen bullying.[3] There was not a significant difference in food allergy incidents between peanut-free schools and schools with peanut-free tables.[3] Beyond the daily lunch activities, other school activities such as field trips, school parties, and after-school activities affect children with food allergies because of potential exposures. Legislation regarding food allergy, encouraging education, and allowing schools to have a stock of epinephrine autoinjectors available are measures that can help children with food allergies attend school in a safe manner.[20,74,75]

Bullying because of food allergies results in increased distress among both children and their parents. Parental interventions regarding bullying have been shown to decrease bullying in children with food allergies, beyond just talking to their child about the incidents. Successful actions that have been associated with decreased bullying included intervening with the help of other adults, such as school personnel or parents of the other child.[76] When bullying remits, quality of life increases. The most effective methods to address bullying include school-based programs that reduce tolerance and increase remediation.[76]

Eating out is a normal social event that can become one of anxiety and stress when families are living with food allergies.[3] When eating out, families must rely on others' knowledge of label reading and cross-contamination issues.[3] Although food workers have generally been noted to be knowledgeable and have positive attitudes regarding food accommodating food allergies, 10% believed that persons with food allergies could still safely consume a small amount of allergen.[13,77] In one study, peanut allergic children reported a greater need to be careful about eating and more anxiety regarding eating compared with diabetic children.[78]

Although most of the burdens fall on the patient, the entire family can often feel the troubles. Everyday tasks such as grocery shopping become time-consuming and expensive to ensure safe and nutritious foods.[3] Caregivers can develop anxiety and an increased sense of protectiveness, especially out of fear for severe reactions and lack of control.[3] Social events such as family gatherings, restaurant outings, parties, travel, and even school become overwhelming when constantly monitoring for allergens and are limited by the food selections at events.[3]

The social-emotional development of a child can be affected by food allergies. When children are unable to participate in social activities such as sleepovers, playing at friends' houses, and other parties, they miss the opportunity to build relationships, solidify friendships, develop autonomy, and improve independence. For those who experience long-standing restrictions, there can be an increase in social isolation and resultant feelings of depression or social anxiety.[3]

CLINICS CARE POINTS

- In IgE-mediated food allergies symptoms present within minutes to no more than 2 hours.
- Symptoms can be seen in multiple organ systems (cutaneous, respiratory, gastrointestinal, and cardiovascular).
- Epinephrine IM is the first-line treatment of anaphylaxis and should not be delayed.
- The most common food allergens are milk, egg, peanut, tree nuts, wheat, soy, fish, and shellfish. Patients with significant pollen sensitization can present with oral symptoms

caused by fresh fruits and vegetables due to pollen-fruit cross-reactivity (pollen-food allergy syndrome).

- Delayed introduction of peanut in children with severe atopic dermatitis and/or egg allergy increases the risk of developing a peanut allergy.
- Diagnosis of food allergy is based on clinical history of past reactions, skin, and blood testing as well as oral food challenges, if applicable.
- Indiscriminate IgE food panel testing has been associated with unnecessary food elimination diets and should be avoided.
- Avoidance of the inciting food is the mainstay of management.
- Oral immunotherapy, sublingual immunotherapy, and epicutaneous immunotherapy are under investigation. The current treatment goal is to achieve sustained unresponsiveness.
- Currently no cure for food allergy exists.
- Food allergy and food avoidance can have a negative impact on quality of life.

DISCLOSURE

The authors have nothing to disclose.

REFERENCES

1. Sicherer SH, Sampson HA. Food allergy: A review and update on epidemiology, pathogenesis, diagnosis, prevention, and management. J Allergy Clin Immunol 2018;141(1):41–58.
2. Osborne NJ, Koplin JJ, Martin PE, et al. Prevalence of challenge-proven IgE-mediated food allergy using population-based sampling and predetermined challenge criteria in infants. J Allergy Clin Immunol 2011;127(3):668–76, e1-2.
3. Bollinger ME, Dahlquist LM, Mudd K, et al. The impact of food allergy on the daily activities of children and their families. Ann Allergy Asthma Immunol 2006;96(3):415–21.
4. Bock SA, Muñoz-Furlong A, Sampson HA. Fatalities due to anaphylactic reactions to foods. J Allergy Clin Immunol. Jan 2001;107(1):191–3.
5. Savage J, Johns CB. Food allergy: epidemiology and natural history. Immunol Allergy Clin North Am 2015;35(1):45–59.
6. Nwaru BI, Hickstein L, Panesar SS, et al. Prevalence of common food allergies in Europe: a systematic review and meta-analysis. Allergy 2014;69(8):992–1007.
7. Poulos LM, Waters AM, Correll PK, et al. Trends in hospitalizations for anaphylaxis, angioedema, and urticaria in Australia, 1993-1994 to 2004-2005. J Allergy Clin Immunol 2007;120(4):878–84.
8. Lin RY, Anderson AS, Shah SN, et al. Increasing anaphylaxis hospitalizations in the first 2 decades of life: New York State, 1990 -2006. Ann Allergy Asthma Immunol 2008;101(4):387–93.
9. Soller L, Ben-Shoshan M, Harrington DW, et al. Overall prevalence of self-reported food allergy in Canada. J Allergy Clin Immunol 2012;130(4):986–8.
10. National Academies of Sciences Eg, and Medicine, Division HaM, Board FaN, Committee on Food Allergies: Global Burden C, Treatment, P.evention, and Public Policy. Finding a Path to Safety in Food Allergy: Assessment of the Global Burden, Causes, Prevention, Management, and Public Policy. 2016.
11. Sicherer SH, Allen K, Lack G, et al. Critical Issues in Food Allergy: A National Academies Consensus Report. Pediatrics 2017;140(2). https://doi.org/10.1542/peds.2017-0194.

12. Prescott SL, Pawankar R, Allen KJ, et al. A global survey of changing patterns of food allergy burden in children. World Allergy Organ J 2013;6(1):21.

13. Anvari S, Miller J, Yeh CY, et al. IgE-Mediated Food Allergy. Clin Rev Allergy Immunol 2019;57(2):244–60.

14. McDole JR, Wheeler LW, McDonald KG, et al. Goblet cells deliver luminal antigen to CD103+ dendritic cells in the small intestine. Nature 2012;483(7389):345–9.

15. Steinbach EC, Plevy SE. The role of macrophages and dendritic cells in the initiation of inflammation in IBD. Inflamm Bowel Dis 2014;20(1):166–75.

16. Coombes JL, Siddiqui KR, Arancibia-Cárcamo CV, et al. A functionally specialized population of mucosal CD103+ DCs induces Foxp3+ regulatory T cells via a TGF-beta and retinoic acid-dependent mechanism. J Exp Med 2007; 204(8):1757–64.

17. Noval Rivas M, Burton OT, Oettgen HC, et al. IL-4 production by group 2 innate lymphoid cells promotes food allergy by blocking regulatory T-cell function. J Allergy Clin Immunol 2016;138(3):801–11.e9.

18. Sehra S, Yao W, Nguyen ET, et al. TH9 cells are required for tissue mast cell accumulation during allergic inflammation. J Allergy Clin Immunol 2015;136(2): 433–40.e1.

19. Koplin JJ, Allen KJ, Gurrin LC, et al. The impact of family history of allergy on risk of food allergy: a population-based study of infants. Int J Environ Res Public Health 2013;10(11):5364–77.

20. Sicherer SH, Sampson HA. Food allergy: Epidemiology, pathogenesis, diagnosis, and treatment. J Allergy Clin Immunol 2014;133(2):291–307, quiz 308.

21. Gupta RS, Walkner MM, Greenhawt M, et al. Food Allergy Sensitization and Presentation in Siblings of Food Allergic Children. J Allergy Clin Immunol Pract 2016; 4(5):956–62.

22. Keet CA, Savage JH, Seopaul S, et al. Temporal trends and racial/ethnic disparity in self-reported pediatric food allergy in the United States. Ann Allergy Asthma Immunol 2014;112(3):222–9.e3.

23. McGowan EC, Keet CA. Prevalence of self-reported food allergy in the National Health and Nutrition Examination Survey (NHANES) 2007-2010. J Allergy Clin Immunol 2013;132(5):1216–9.e5.

24. Gupta RS, Springston EE, Warrier MR, et al. The prevalence, severity, and distribution of childhood food allergy in the United States. Pediatrics 2011;128(1): e9–17.

25. Liu AH, Jaramillo R, Sicherer SH, et al. National prevalence and risk factors for food allergy and relationship to asthma: results from the National Health and Nutrition Examination Survey 2005-2006. J Allergy Clin Immunol 2010;126(4): 798–806.e13.

26. Du Toit G, Roberts G, Sayre PH, et al. Identifying infants at high risk of peanut allergy: the Learning Early About Peanut Allergy (LEAP) screening study. J Allergy Clin Immunol 2013;131(1):135–43, e1-e12.

27. Keet CA, Wood RA, Matsui EC. Personal and parental nativity as risk factors for food sensitization. J Allergy Clin Immunol 2012;129(1):169–75, e1-5.

28. Seth D, Poowutikul P, Pansare M, et al. Food Allergy: A Review. Pediatr Ann 2020; 49(1):e50–8.

29. Savage JH, Lee-Sarwar KA, Sordillo J, et al. A prospective microbiome-wide association study of food sensitization and food allergy in early childhood. Allergy 2018;73(1):145–52.

30. Upton J, Nowak-Wegrzyn A. The Impact of Baked Egg and Baked Milk Diets on IgE- and Non-IgE-Mediated Allergy. Clin Rev Allergy Immunol 2018;55(2): 118–38.
31. Martin PE, Eckert JK, Koplin JJ, et al. Which infants with eczema are at risk of food allergy? Results from a population-based cohort. Clin Exp Allergy 2015; 45(1):255–64.
32. Sharma HP, Bansil S, Uygungil B. Signs and Symptoms of Food Allergy and Food-Induced Anaphylaxis. Pediatr Clin North Am 2015;62(6):1377–92.
33. Ho MH, Wong WH, Chang C. Clinical spectrum of food allergies: a comprehensive review. Clin Rev Allergy Immunol 2014;46(3):225–40.
34. Gupta RS, Springston EE, Kim JS, et al. Food allergy knowledge, attitudes, and beliefs of primary care physicians. Pediatrics 2010;125(1):126–32.
35. Franxman TJ, Howe L, Teich E, et al. Oral food challenge and food allergy quality of life in caregivers of children with food allergy. J Allergy Clin Immunol Pract 2015;3(1):50–6.
36. Muraro A, Werfel T, Hoffmann-Sommergruber K, et al. EAACI food allergy and anaphylaxis guidelines: diagnosis and management of food allergy. Allergy 2014;69(8):1008–25.
37. Ocmant A, Mulier S, Hanssens L, et al. Basophil activation tests for the diagnosis of food allergy in children. Clin Exp Allergy 2009;39(8):1234–45.
38. Santos AF, Douiri A, Bécares N, et al. Basophil activation test discriminates between allergy and tolerance in peanut-sensitized children. J Allergy Clin Immunol 2014;134(3):645–52.
39. Sicherer SH, Wood RA, Vickery BP, et al. Impact of Allergic Reactions on Food-Specific IgE Concentrations and Skin Test Results. J Allergy Clin Immunol Pract 2016;4(2):239–45.e4.
40. Nowak-Wegrzyn A, Assa'ad AH, Bahna SL, et al. Work Group report: oral food challenge testing. J Allergy Clin Immunol 2009;123(6 Suppl):S365–83.
41. Sampson HA, Gerth van Wijk R, Bindslev-Jensen C, et al. Standardizing double-blind, placebo-controlled oral food challenges: American Academy of Allergy, Asthma & Immunology-European Academy of Allergy and Clinical Immunology PRACTALL consensus report. J Allergy Clin Immunol 2012;130(6):1260–74.
42. Bernstein IL, Li JT, Bernstein DI, et al. Allergy diagnostic testing: an updated practice parameter. Ann Allergy Asthma Immunol 2008;100(3 Suppl 3):S1–148.
43. Saarinen KM, Suomalainen H, Savilahti E. Diagnostic value of skin-prick and patch tests and serum eosinophil cationic protein and cow's milk-specific IgE in infants with cow's milk allergy. Clin Exp Allergy 2001;31(3):423–9.
44. Boyano-Martínez T, García-Ara C, Díaz-Pena JM, et al. Prediction of tolerance on the basis of quantification of egg white-specific IgE antibodies in children with egg allergy. J Allergy Clin Immunol 2002;110(2):304–9.
45. Wang J, Godbold JH, Sampson HA. Correlation of serum allergy (IgE) tests performed by different assay systems. J Allergy Clin Immunol 2008;121(5):1219–24.
46. Boyce JA, Assa'ad A, Burks AW, et al. Guidelines for the Diagnosis and Management of Food Allergy in the United States: Summary of the NIAID-Sponsored Expert Panel Report. J Allergy Clin Immunol 2010;126(6):1105–18.
47. Hourihane JO, Dean TP, Warner JO. Peanut allergy in relation to heredity, maternal diet, and other atopic diseases: results of a questionnaire survey, skin prick testing, and food challenges. BMJ 1996;313(7056):518–21.
48. Poncet P, Sénéchal H, Charpin D. Update on pollen-food allergy syndrome. Expert Rev Clin Immunol 2020;16(6):561–78.

49. Sicherer SH, Simons FE, Section on Allergy and Immunology AeAoP. Self-inject-able epinephrine for first-aid management of anaphylaxis. Pediatrics 2007; 119(3):638–46.

50. Marrs T, Lack G. Why do few food-allergic adolescents treat anaphylaxis with adrenaline?–Reviewing a pressing issue. Pediatr Allergy Immunol 2013;24(3): 222–9.

51. Shemesh E, D'Urso C, Knight C, et al. Food-Allergic Adolescents at Risk for Anaphylaxis: A Randomized Controlled Study of Supervised Injection to Improve Comfort with Epinephrine Self-Injection. J Allergy Clin Immunol Pract 2017;5(2): 391–7.e4.

52. Fleming JT, Clark S, Camargo CA, et al. Early treatment of food-induced anaphy-laxis with epinephrine is associated with a lower risk of hospitalization. J Allergy Clin Immunol Pract 2015;3(1):57–62.

53. Simons FE, Simons KJ. Histamine and H1-antihistamines: celebrating a century of progress. J Allergy Clin Immunol 2011;128(6):1139–50.e4.

54. Karam M, Scherzer R, Ogbogu PU, et al. Food allergy prevalence, knowledge, and behavioral trends among college students - A 6-year comparison. J Allergy Clin Immunol Pract 2017;5(2):504–6.e5.

55. Shaker M, Bean K, Verdi M. Economic evaluation of epinephrine auto-injectors for peanut allergy. Ann Allergy Asthma Immunol 2017;119(2):160–3.

56. David TJ, Waddington E, Stanton RH. Nutritional hazards of elimination diets in children with atopic eczema. Arch Dis Child 1984;59(4):323–5.

57. Sova C, Feuling MB, Baumler M, et al. Systematic review of nutrient intake and growth in children with multiple IgE-mediated food allergies. Nutr Clin Pract 2013;28(6):669–75.

58. Anagnostou K, Islam S, King Y, et al. Assessing the efficacy of oral immuno-therapy for the desensitisation of peanut allergy in children (STOP II): a phase 2 randomised controlled trial. Lancet 2014;383(9925):1297–304.

59. Jones SM, Sicherer SH, Burks AW, et al. Epicutaneous immunotherapy for the treatment of peanut allergy in children and young adults. J Allergy Clin Immunol 2017;139(4):1242–52.e9.

60. Narisety SD, Frischmeyer-Guerrerio PA, Keet CA, et al. A randomized, double-blind, placebo-controlled pilot study of sublingual versus oral immunotherapy for the treatment of peanut allergy. J Allergy Clin Immunol 2015;135(5): 1275–82, e1-6.

61. Sampson HA, Leung DY, Burks AW, et al. A phase II, randomized, double-blind, parallel-group, placebo-controlled oral food challenge trial of Xolair (omalizumab) in peanut allergy. J Allergy Clin Immunol 2011;127(5):1309–13010.e1.

62. Grohskopf LA, Sokolow LZ, Broder KR, et al. Prevention and Control of Seasonal Influenza with Vaccines: Recommendations of the Advisory Committee on Immu-nization Practices - United States, 2017-18 Influenza Season. MMWR Recomm Rep (Morb Mortal Wkly Rep) 2017;66(2):1–20.

63. Greenhawt M, Turner PJ, Kelso JM. Administration of influenza vaccines to egg allergic recipients: A practice parameter update 2017. Ann Allergy Asthma Im-munol 2018;120(1):49–52.

64. Cetron MS, Marfin AA, Julian KG, et al. Yellow fever vaccine. Recommendations of the Advisory Committee on Immunization Practices (ACIP). MMWR Recomm Rep (Morb Mortal Wkly Rep) 2002;51(RR-17):1–11 ; quiz CE1-4.

65. Roduit C, Frei R, Depner M, et al. Increased food diversity in the first year of life is inversely associated with allergic diseases. J Allergy Clin Immunol 2014;133(4): 1056–64.

66. Du Toit G, Roberts G, Sayre PH, et al. Randomized trial of peanut consumption in infants at risk for peanut allergy. N Engl J Med 2015;372(9):803–13.
67. Greer FR, Sicherer SH, Burks AW, et al. Effects of early nutritional interventions on the development of atopic disease in infants and children: the role of maternal dietary restriction, breastfeeding, timing of introduction of complementary foods, and hydrolyzed formulas. Pediatrics 2008;121(1):183–91.
68. Fleischer DM, Spergel JM, Assa'ad AH, et al. Primary prevention of allergic disease through nutritional interventions. J Allergy Clin Immunol Pract 2013;1(1): 29–36.
69. Onizawa Y, Noguchi E, Okada M, et al. The Association of the Delayed Introduction of Cow's Milk with IgE-Mediated Cow's Milk Allergies. J Allergy Clin Immunol Pract 2016;4(3):481–8.e2.
70. Allen KJ, Koplin JJ, Ponsonby AL, et al. Vitamin D insufficiency is associated with challenge-proven food allergy in infants. J Allergy Clin Immunol 2013;131(4): 1109–16.
71. Simpson EL, Chalmers JR, Hanifin JM, et al. Emollient enhancement of the skin barrier from birth offers effective atopic dermatitis prevention. J Allergy Clin Immunol 2014;134(4):818–23.
72. Horimukai K, Morita K, Narita M, et al. Application of moisturizer to neonates prevents development of atopic dermatitis. J Allergy Clin Immunol 2014;134(4): 824–30.e6.
73. Bartnikas LM, Huffaker MF, Sheehan WJ, et al. Impact of school peanut-free policies on epinephrine administration. J Allergy Clin Immunol 2017;140(2):465–73.
74. Szychlinski C, Schmeissing KA, Fuleihan Z, et al. Food allergy emergency preparedness in Illinois schools: rural disparity in guideline implementation. J Allergy Clin Immunol Pract 2015;3(5):805–7.e8.
75. White L, Aubin J, Bradford C, et al. Effectiveness of a computer module to augment the training of school staff in the management of students with food allergies. Ann Allergy Asthma Immunol 2015;114(3):254–5.e3.
76. Annunziato RA, Rubes M, Ambrose MA, et al. Longitudinal evaluation of food allergy-related bullying. J Allergy Clin Immunol Pract 2014;2(5):639–41.
77. Radke TJ, Brown LG, Hoover ER, et al. Food Allergy Knowledge and Attitudes of Restaurant Managers and Staff: An EHS-Net Study. J Food Prot 2016;79(9): 1588–98.
78. Avery NJ, King RM, Knight S, et al. Assessment of quality of life in children with peanut allergy. Pediatr Allergy Immunol 2003;14(5):378–82.

Penicillin Allergy
Mechanisms, Diagnosis, and Management

Estelle A. Green, BS[a], Kelan Fogarty, BS[a],
Faoud T. Ishmael, MD, PhD[a,b,*]

KEYWORDS

• Penicillin allergy • Hypersensitivity • Skin testing • Drug challenge • Desensitization

KEY POINTS

• Penicillin allergy is common and can occur through multiple types of hypersensitivity mechanisms.
• History and physical examination are key to evaluation of penicillin allergy.
• Penicillin allergy is most often lost over time.
• Allergy skin testing and/or drug provocation challenge can accurately diagnose penicillin allergy.

INTRODUCTION

The discovery of penicillin in 1928 by Sir Alexander Fleming changed the course of modern medicine. Once fatal diseases such as sepsis, meningitis, and endocarditis could now be cured. Penicillins have saved countless lives since then and continue to be the first-line treatment of many infectious diseases. It is still the only recommended treatment of prevention of mother-to-child transmission of syphilis. However, allergic reactions are common, and the first case of anaphylaxis was reported in 1945.[1]

The prevalence of penicillin allergy in the United States is approximately 10%.[2] In part, this is driven by the high rate of use of this drug because the vast majority of the population has received this antibiotic (often multiple times by adulthood). The chemical nature of penicillin also plays a large role in susceptibility to allergic reactions. The carbonyl group of the beta-lactam ring is an excellent electrophile (**Fig. 1**, labeled *), which provides the ability to covalently bind to proteins and is the basis for its ability to block bacterial cell wall synthesis by inhibiting bacterial transpeptidase. However, this also allows the drug to act as a hapten, by covalently binding to

[a] Pennsylvania State University, College of Medicine University Park, 1850 East Park Avenue, State College, PA 16803, USA; [b] Mount Nittany Health, 1850 East Park Avenue, State College, PA 16803, USA
* Corresponding author. 1850 East Park Avenue, Suite 201, State College, PA 16803.
E-mail address: faoud.ishmael@mountnittany.org

Prim Care Clin Office Pract 50 (2023) 221–235
https://doi.org/10.1016/j.pop.2022.11.002
0095-4543/23/© 2022 Elsevier Inc. All rights reserved.
primarycare.theclinics.com

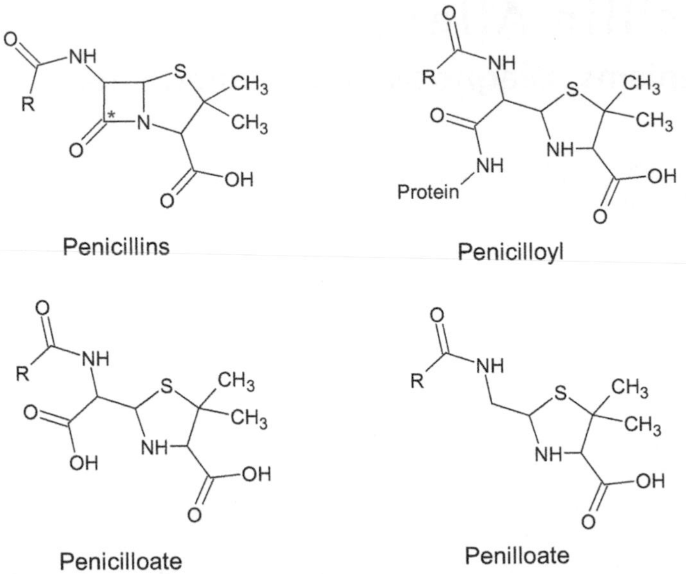

Fig. 1. Chemical structure of penicillins. Asterix indicates carbonyl group that is the site of covalent bond to carrier protein. Penicilloyl is the major determinant of allergic reactions. The penicillin ring can isomerize into minor determinants (penicilloate and penilloate) that less commonly cause reactions.

circulating proteins (carriers) and forming a neoantigen that looks foreign to the immune system.

Drug allergies occur across a spectrum of reaction severities that range from benign rashes to life-threatening reactions. Some reactions warrant lifelong avoidance of the allergenic medication, while the drug may be safely used again in other cases. As a result, it is important to develop a framework to not only manage acute reactions, but to determine when it is appropriate to test for drug allergies, when to use an allergenic medication again, and when it is appropriate to refer to an allergist.

For many years, our approach to penicillin allergy was to simply have drug-allergic patients avoid the medication, often lifelong. However, recent data in the past few years have demonstrated potential harm in doing this. First, only about 10% of the population with a penicillin allergy listed on chart is actually allergic.[2] The majority of patients (~80%) lose their penicillin allergy during a 5 to 10-year period.[2] Second, many patients with a chart listing of penicillin allergy may not have been allergic to begin with. In some cases, they could have had a viral exanthem or idiopathic urticaria that was blamed on the medication. In other cases, patients developed side effects (eg, vomiting and diarrhea) that were recorded as allergies.

There are significant consequences to needlessly avoiding penicillin. As penicillin is still the first-line treatment of many infections, penicillin-allergic patients may receive second-line medications that are less effective. This could result in more treatment failures, infections that are more difficult to treat, and longer hospital stays.[3-5] Moreover, patients with penicillin allergy may receive stronger antibiotics or those with broader spectrum than would be needed for their infection. Patients with penicillin allergy are more likely to receive IV antibiotics in the hospital, have higher utilization of vancomycin, and as a result, more likely to develop vancomycin-resistant enterococcus.[6,7] We and others also demonstrated that penicillin-allergic patients were more likely to develop difficult-to-treat infections such as methicillin-resistant *Staphylococcus aureus* and *Clostridium difficile*, possibly due to receiving nonpenicillin, broad-spectrum antibiotics.[4,5,7] Macy and Shu demonstrated that removing the penicillin allergy label decreased outpatient visits, ER visits, and days of hospitalization.[3] Moreover, these patients were exposed to less clindamycin and macrolides during future hospital stays.[3]

Health-care cost may be significantly higher for penicillin-allergic patients. In the Kaiser Permanente system, penicillin allergy was associated with 30,433 additional hospital days during a 3-year period, resulting in more than US$64 million in additional health-care expenditures.[7] A recent study sought to determine financial benefits of penicillin testing. They determined that penicillin allergy testing (combining data from United States and Europe) would reduce inpatient costs by US$657 per patient (US$1440 in United States and US$489 in Europe) and outpatient costs by US$2476 (US$256 in United States and US$6045 in Europe).[8]

It is therefore beneficial to accurately determine whether a patient truly has a penicillin allergy because this has significant influence on current and future management of infections, health-care utilization, and health-care costs. This review article will focus on the clinical presentation of penicillin hypersensitivity reactions and their acute management, in addition to approaches to diagnosis and clearing penicillin allergy when appropriate. These approaches will include those that can be performed in the primary care office as well as those for which referral to an allergist would be indicated. Although this review focuses on managing patients with penicillin allergy, this approach can be extended to almost any other drug allergy.

MECHANISMS OF PENICILLIN ALLERGY
Type I Immediate Hypersensitivity (IgE-Mediated)

Type I hypersensitivity, or immediate reactions, are mediated by IgE antibodies in response to proteins perceived as foreign by the immune system. Although lone penicillin molecules are too small to drive an immunologic antibody response, they can covalently bind to proteins in plasma and form immunogenic hapten–carrier complexes.[9] The most common hapten, penicilloyl (see **Fig. 1**), is created when the penicillin beta-lactam ring covalently binds to common serum proteins' lysine residues. Penicilloyl, also called the "major determinant," is responsible for 60% to 85% of penicillin reactions.[10,11] Additionally, penicillin can isomerize and form other hapten complexes such as penicilloate and penilloate (see **Fig. 1**). These molecules are also known as "minor determinants" and account for 10% to 20% of penicillin allergies.[10] Reactions to minor determinants are more often associated with anaphylaxis as opposed to the major determinant. Ultimately, the penicillin moiety (hapten) and protein (carrier) form a neoantigen—"new" antigen that is recognized as foreign by the immune system (**Fig. 2**). The penicillin hapten–carrier protein is taken up by antigen-presenting cells (APCs), such as dendritic cells, and presented to naive CD4+ T cells through MHC-II complexes in lymph nodes, which results in type 2 helper T (Th2) cell differentiation. Th2 cells then induce the differentiation and isotype switching of naive B cells into plasma cells producing IgE antibodies specific to the penicillin hapten–carrier complex. These IgE bind to the constant region (Fc) of epsilon receptors on the surface of basophils and mast cells, which will subsequently activate on reexposure.[1,10] Because this sensitization process typically takes weeks, patients are generally asymptomatic during the last course of penicillin.[10] On reexposure of the drug, hapten–carrier complexes activate basophils and mast cells by binding to IgE, which cross-links the Fc epsilon receptors and induces the degranulation of

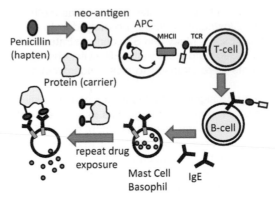

Fig. 2. IgE-mediated drug allergy. Penicillin (hapten) covalently binds to a circulating protein (carrier), forming a neo-antigen. This is taken up by APC, processed, and presented to CD4+T-cells via the MHCII complex. T-cells then stimulate B-cells that have antibodies specific to the neoantigen, leading to IgE production. The IgE then binds to mast cells and basophils. On repeat exposure to penicillin, the IgE on mast cells/basophils bind the neo-antigen, triggering allergic mediator release, which produces the clinical symptoms of an allergic reaction.

basophils and mast cells. The release of inflammatory mediators such as tryptase, histamine, prostaglandins, and leukotrienes drive the clinical manifestation of type 1 hypersensitivity, which includes urticaria, angioedema, bronchospasm, gastrointestinal symptoms (abdominal pain, nausea, vomiting, diarrhea), cardiovascular collapse, and anaphylaxis. These symptoms typically have an onset of minutes to hours following reexposure.[10] Because penicillin-specific IgE antibodies decrease over time, patients with past reactions may lose sensitivity following a period of avoidance. In fact, ~50% of patients with IgE-mediated penicillin can lose the sensitivity after 5 years; this increases to 80% after 10 years.[12–14]

Type II Cytotoxic Hypersensitivity (IgM and IgG-Mediated)

Type II hypersensitivity, or cytotoxic reactions, are mediated by IgM or IgG antibodies binding to cellular surface antigens. Major and minor penicillin determinants covalently bind to cell surface proteins (typically on white blood cells, red blood cells, or platelets) and together, they act as antigens. IgG, or less commonly IgM, is the predominant antibody involved in this type of reaction. When exposed to penicillin, the preformed antibodies bind to the penicillin-surface protein complexes and induce cellular destruction via complement activation and/or phagocytosis by macrophages, leading to hemolytic anemia (as the case illustrated above), neutropenia, or thrombocytopenia.[15] Typical onset is 1 week to months after drug initiation. Although reactions typically resolve after penicillin discontinuation, symptoms can develop within hours after reexposure because IgM and IgG antibodies can persist for years.[15,16] It is therefore crucial to avoid the drug permanently.

Type III Immunocomplex Hypersensitivity

Type III hypersensitivity, or immune complex reactions, are mediated by immune complexes consisting of a soluble antigen (ie, circulating protein) bound by an antibody. A similar hapten–carrier as discussed above generates IgG or IgM antibodies. Binding of these antibodies to the penicillin-soluble protein leads to immune complex formation, which can deposit in tissues (blood vessels, kidneys, and joints). The penicillin–IgG complex then activates the complement system, which releases chemotactic agents that recruit inflammatory cells (neutrophils and macrophages). These inflammatory cells release lysosomal enzymes and free radicals causing inflammatory tissue damage. Symptoms can vary with the site of the penicillin–IgG complex deposition. Namely, complexes deposited in blood vessels, kidneys, and joints, will result in urticarial, vasculitis, nephritis, and arthritis, respectively. Symptoms typically occur 1 to 3 weeks after drug initiation since a significant quantity of antibodies is required to generate this type of reaction, which takes weeks to be produced.[17,18]

Type IV Delayed Cell-Mediated Hypersensitivity

Type IV hypersensitivity, also known as cell-mediated or delayed reactions, are mediated by CD4+ (helper) and CD8+ (killer) T-cells. There are 4 subtypes of delayed reaction that are characterized by the effector cells involved and clinical phenotypes (**Fig. 3**): Type IVa (Th1 helper T-cell and macrophages), Type IVb (Th2 helper T-cell and eosinophils), Type IVc (CD8+), and Type IVd (CD8+, Th17 helper T-cell and neutrophils).[10] They all consist of a sensitization (exposure leading to activation of allergic cells) followed by an elicitation phase (allergic cells producing the reaction). There are 2 proposed hypotheses for the sensitization phase: the hapten model and the "p-""(primary interaction) model.[19] In the hapten model, penicillin haptens bind to self-proteins and form a penicillin protein–hapten complex that is taken up and proteolytically processed by APCs, and presented on MHC to T-cells specific to the penicillin hapten–protein complex. In the p-i model, penicillin directly binds to T-cell receptors and MHC protein (p-i HLA) without the need for covalently binding to a protein. This directly activates T-cells leading to differentiation of helper and effector T-cells.[19-21] In both models, CD4+ T-cells stimulate other cells (eg, macrophages, eosinophils, neutrophils), which lead to tissue damage, and/or CD8+ T-cells induce apoptosis in cells.[19]

TYPE IVa

Type IVa hypersensitivity is mediated by a Th1 helper T-cell immune response resulting in macrophage activation. The sensitization phase involves priming of Th1 cells (via the hapten or p-i model). During the elicitation phase, Th1 cells are recruited to the skin

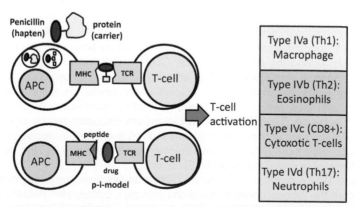

Fig. 3. Type IV drug hypersensitivity. T-cells can be stimulated via 2 pathways, presentation by APC of penicillin-covalently linked to a protein, or direct interaction of penicillin with a T-cell receptor and MHC (p-i model). T-cells may differentiate via 4 main pathways (Type IVa–d), which produce different cellular responses and distinct drug hypersensitivity conditions.

where they secrete inflammatory cytokines (mainly IFN-γ and TNF-α) leading to macrophage activation and inflammatory response.[10,20] The typical rash is either macular or maculopapular. These generally occur 1 to 2 weeks following initial drug exposure and commonly manifest toward the end of a course of penicillins. If someone receives a subsequent course of penicillin, the rash could develop within 24 to 72 hours of reexposure. In general, these reactions tend to be of mild-to-moderate severity and usually go away quickly after the offending drug is removed. This allergy may also be lost quickly, potentially within months. Mill and colleagues[22] demonstrated that 94.1% of children challenged after this type of drug allergy are able to tolerate it without any reactions.

TYPE IVb

Type IVb hypersensitivities are mediated by Th2 immune response resulting in eosinophilic activation. The sensitization phase involves priming of Th2 cells. During the elicitation phase, Th2-cells secrete IL-5, which is a potent cytokine that drives eosinophil proliferation and survival. Eosinophils traffic to diverse tissues, including skin, kidney, liver, in addition to lungs, nervous system, and heart. When activated, eosinophils release cytotoxic granule proteins resulting in systemic inflammation and organ damage.[23]

A clinical syndrome associated with this reaction is drug reaction with eosinophilia and systemic symptoms (DRESS).[23] It has been suggested that B-cell secretion of IL-10 during the sensitization phase may induce viral reactivation and subsequent inappropriate systemic immune response in the context of DRESS. Namely, members of the human herpes viridae family (primarily HHV-6, EBV, and CMV) are thought to trigger uncontrolled T-cell activation. In turn, T-cells release cytokines that drive eosinophilia, leading to systemic inflammation features found in DRESS patients.[23] Symptoms include maculopapular eruption, edema, fever, lymphadenopathy, and systemic organ (more commonly heart, lung, liver, kidney) damage, which can lead to death.[24] They generally occur 2 to 8 weeks after the initiation of penicillin.[25] DRESS is considered a severe, life-threatening rash that requires immediate discontinuation of the culprit drug, hospital admission, and prompt treatment.

TYPE IVc

Type IVc hypersensitivities are mediated by CD8+ T-cells resulting in extensive epithelial cell apoptosis and necrosis. The sensitization phase involves priming of CD8+ T-cells. During the elicitation phase, CD8+ T-cells release cytotoxic proteins (granulysin, perforin, Fas ligand, TNF-α, and IFN-γ) leading to keratinocyte necrosis, ranging from partial to full-thickness necrosis of the epidermis. Clinical syndromes associated with this reaction are Stevens-Johnson syndrome (SJS) and Toxic Epidermal Necrolysis (TEN).[26,27] Both conditions are characterized by significant necrosis and detachment of the epidermis; less than 10% epidermal involvement is classified as SJS, more than 30% epidermal involvement is classified as TEN, and 10% to 30% involvement is classified as SJS/TEN overlap.[10]

In SJS and TEN, a prodrome of fever and influenza-like symptoms may develop 1 to 3 days before the mucocutaneous reactions (vesicles, bullae, skin detachment). Severe epidermal detachment may lead to fluid loss, electrolyte imbalance, sepsis, and multiorgan failure.[26,27] Mucosal involvement is common and patients frequently have oral lesions. Any mucosal surface can be involved, including eyes, lungs, gastrointestinal tract, and genitourinary tract. Generally, symptoms occur 4 days to 4 weeks following drug initiation. SJS and TEN are severe reactions with an overall mortality rate ranging from 10% for SJS to 50% for TEN.[28]

TYPE IVd

Type IVd hypersensitivities are mediated by CD8+ and Th17 immune responses resulting in neutrophilic inflammation. The sensitization phase involves priming of CD8+ and Th17 cells. During the elicitation phase, CD8+ T-cells and Th17 migrate to the skin where they release chemokines (CXCL8, IFN-γ, GM-CSF) leading to neutrophil recruitment and sterile pustule formation.[29–31] A clinical syndrome associated with this reaction is acute generalized exanthematous pustulosis (AGEP). Clinical manifestation includes fever, neutrophilic leukocytosis, erythema, and development of numerous small sterile pustules. Symptoms typically develop within 24 to 48 hours of drug exposure and resolve spontaneously in 1 to 2 week following drug discontinuation.[31]

DISCUSSION
Management of Allergic Reactions

Type I hypersensitivity
Most commonly, urticaria and angioedema are the primary symptoms from IgE-mediated drug allergies, and they typically occur within minutes of drug administration. Although rare, anaphylaxis due to penicillin allergy can occur. The medication should be stopped immediately and treatment should be sought immediately.[32] Anaphylaxis is defined as an allergic reaction that involves multiple organ systems, or a severe reaction involving the cardiovascular or respiratory system. Immediate epinephrine administration, followed by antihistamines, is the key to combating anaphylaxis. . Epinephrine is lifesaving in these circumstances and should be injected intramuscularly into the outer thigh at a concentration of 0.01 mg/kg of body weight, not exceeding 0.5 mg.[33] Administration of epinephrine activates adrenergic receptors that help increase peripheral resistance and cardiac output and can therefore mitigate hypotension and shock.[34,35] Additionally, its administration produces bronchodilation and may inhibit mast cell and basophil release of inflammatory mediators, which help alleviate pulmonary symptoms, such as shortness of breath.[34] The vasoconstrictive effects also help to relieve angioedema and urticaria. Potential adverse events (tachycardia, elevated blood pressure) should be considered especially for individuals at high-risk (eg, elderly and those with comorbidities) but these should not prevent the use of epinephrine.[36,37]

Antihistamines can be used to supplement epinephrine therapy. Antihistamines help resolve cutaneous associations of anaphylaxis (eg, urticaria and pruritus) and can be used with epinephrine or as monotherapy in nonanaphylactic reactions if only the skin is involved (mostly to provide symptomatic comfort).[38–40]

Type II hypersensitivity
Although rare, drug-induced hemolytic anemias to penicillins (and also cephalosporins) are possible.[41–43] The mainstay treatment of drug-induced hemolytic anemia is removal of the causative agent.[41,43–45] Depending on the severity, patients can be given blood transfusions.[43,45] Glucocorticoids have negligible effects on improving the anemia.[44,46,47]

Type III hypersensitivity
Serum sickness or serum sickness-like reactions are typically self-limiting as long as the offending agent is removed.[48] If no contraindication to non-steroidal anti-

inflammatory drugs (NSAIDs) (eg, renal failure, history of NSAID allergy), these can help to symptomatically improve arthralgias. Antihistamines can be considered to treat the rash, although its efficacy has not been studied and may be low. In more severe cases (eg, disabling arthralgias or angioedema), glucocorticoids can be given.[48] Responses may be variable, and in some cases, the symptoms may start to wane in as a little as a day.[48]

Type IV hypersensitivity

Type IVa Reactions: These reactions tend to be primarily cutaneous, typically with a macular or maculopapular rash of varying pruritic intensity that is usually mild-to-moderate severity. There is little published data on optimal regimens but our group utilizes cetirizine 10 mg BID in addition to hydroxyzine 25 to 50 mg at bedtime. These rashes typically self resolve within a few days, and glucocorticoids (0.5 mg/kg) with a tapering dose during 1 week can be considered in cases refractory to antihistamines.

Drug reaction of eosinophilia and systemic symptoms

The mainstay treatment is removal of the offending agent and glucocorticoids.[49] A typical starting dose is 1 mg/kg, with a very slow taper during 1 to 3 months. In refractory cases, higher doses can be used initially, 250 to 500 mg for the first few days, followed by a decrease to 1 mg/kg and then a slow taper. In refractory cases, cyclosporine can be considered.[25,49]

Stevens-Johnsons syndrome and toxic epidermal necrolysis

Immediate removal of the causative agent is the first step. These disorders can involve dramatic loss of skin barrier, and patients typically need to be transferred to a burn center. It is imperative to initiate this as quick as possible. Patients are susceptible to damage of any mucosal surface—ocular, oral, gastrointestinal, genitourinary; hence, these all need to be considered. It is essential to consult ophthalmology to perform a slit lamp eye examination (even if the patient has no ocular complaints) because these reactions can produce corneal scarring and blindness. Supportive therapy is also recommended to achieve proper fluid, nutritional, pain, and oxygenation statuses.[50–52] Skin assessment and antibiotic treatment of infections should be performed.[53,54] Several different treatments have been proposed: glucocorticoids, IVIG, cyclosporine, plasmapheresis, and TNF inhibitor.[54] However, data is inconclusive. Glucocorticoids may increase mortality, particularly later in the course of the reaction, so these are generally avoided. IVIG in high doses (2 g/kg given over 2 days) may be beneficial.[55]

Acute generalized exanthematous pustulosis. Mainly, AGEP will resolve on its own once the inciting agent is removed, although supportive therapy (eg, emollients, keeping the skin dry and clean) can be used.[56] Glucocorticoids have not been shown to be useful.[57–59]

Treating through a penicillin rash

Cutaneous manifestations are the most common manifestation of an allergic reaction to penicillin. In cases of mild-to-moderate drug reactions (most often Type IVa), there are indications where the allergenic medication may be continued despite the reaction. This would most often be considered in cases of moderate-to-severe infections when an alternative medication is not an option. In these cases, the antibiotic can be continued, and the patient treated with antihistamines as described above. Cetirizine 10 mg BID ± hydroxyzine 25 mg QHS ± prednisone 20 to 40 mg daily (depending on severity of the initial reaction).

Potential cross-reactivity of other antimicrobials

Historically, there is thought to be approximately 5% to 10% cross-reactivity between penicillins and cephalosporins (mostly with first-generation and second-generation cephalosporins) but the majority of patients with a penicillin allergy can tolerate cephalosporins.[60]

A prudent approach in penicillin-allergic patients is to avoid first-generation or second–generation cephalosporins, or cephalosporins with side chains similar to penicillins **(Table 1)**.[61] There is not significant cross-reactivity with monobactams, and these are safe to use in penicillin-allergic patients.[61] Cross-reactivity with carbapenems is low, approximately 1%, so these can also be safely used.[62]

Diagnostic Testing for Penicillin Allergy

Skin testing

Penicillin skin testing should be done by personnel who are trained to interpret results and treat allergic reactions. In recent years, there has been an effort to train pharmacists and infection control groups to perform testing. Skin testing for penicillin is a highly sensitive test to evaluate IgE-mediated allergy.[2]

Skin testing with the major determinant (ie, penicilloyl polylysine, commercially available as PRE-PEN) and penicillin G is approximately 95% sensitive. A positive and negative control should be utilized (histamine and saline, respectively).[2] Initially, a skin prick to each of these is performed in duplicate, followed by intradermal testing if the former is negative. A positive test is a wheal that is 3 mm greater than the negative control. When the skin test is negative, an oral challenge to penicillin (250–500 mg) is performed, and the combination of the two is close to 100% sensitive to detect IgE-mediated reactions.[63–65] The positive predictive value is estimated to be 40% to 100%; therefore, given the potential of false-positive tests, penicillin testing is not recommended as a screening test; it should only be done to determine whether the allergy is still present in patients with a history of reaction.[63,65,66]

Patch testing

Patch testing may be performed to test for Type IV reactions. This is administered using a 5% or 10% concentration of penicillin in petroleum jelly (weight/volume) applied to the skin in a Finn chamber, worn for 48 hours, and is read 15 minutes after removal and again 24 hours after removal.[67] The specificity is high, approaching 100%, although the sensitivity is lower, approximately 50%.[68,69]

Table 1
Beta-lactam antibiotics with similar side chains

Amoxicillin	Ampicillin	Ceftraixone	Cefoxitin	Cefamandole	Ceftazidime
Cefadroxil	Cefaclor	Cefotaxime	Cephaloridine	Cefonicid	Aztreonam
Cefprozil	Cephalexin	Cefpodoxime	Cephalothin		
Cefatrizine	Cephradine	Cefditoren			
	Cephaloglycin	Ceftizoxime			
	Loracarbef	Cefmenoxime			

Each column represents drugs with identical R1 side chains.
From Joint Task Force on Practice Parameters; American Academy of Allergy, Asthma and Immunology; American College of Allergy, Asthma and Immunology; Joint Council of Allergy, Asthma and Immunology. Drug allergy: an updated practice parameter. Ann Allergy Asthma Immunol. 2010;105(4):259-273.

Blood testing

There is no role for blood work in diagnosing IgE-mediated reactions. Although IgE assays for penicillin exist, these have poor sensitivity and specificity. Blood tests may be of utility in type II hypersensitivity reactions. A modified Coombs test can be used to confirm a drug reaction, by adding the culprit drug to patient blood during the assay. Blood testing may also be helpful in type III reactions. Often C3 and C4 levels are low due to complement consumption, and measuring kidney and liver function and inflammatory markers can help to assess the severity of reaction.

Blood testing can also be useful in Type IV reactions. In DRESS, blood eosinophils are typically 1500 cells/mcl or greater, and there is often liver or renal dysfunction. Although blood testing cannot be used to diagnose other Type IV reactions, it can help to assess severity by determining whether organ dysfunction is present.

Skin biopsy. Skin biopsies are not helpful to diagnose Type I or Type II hypersensitivity reactions and have a low diagnostic yield in Type III reactions. Skin biopsies are most helpful in diagnosing Type IVc reactions (SJS/TEN) because it can help to exclude several other rashes that may be in the differential (eg, bullous linear IgA dermatosis, autoimmune bullous skin conditions, scalded skin syndrome).

Graded challenge

The graded challenge is the gold standard of IgE testing, and involves administering a medication systemically (oral or injected).[2] This is done when the pretest probability of a true allergy is low. For oral medications, 10% of the therapeutic dose is given and the individual observed for 30 to 60 minutes. If someone were allergic, this dose is usually low enough that the reaction would be mild. Assuming no reaction, then 90% of the therapeutic dose is given with observation for 30 to 60 minutes. For intravenous medications where (there may be risk of a more severe reaction), the starting dose is often 1% of therapeutic dose, then 10%, and 100% with 30 minutes of observation between each dose.

There are instances where type IV hypersensitivity reactions can be evaluated with a graded challenge. In these scenarios, the 10%/90% protocol from above is implemented because some Type IV reactions may occur within an hour due to the presence of memory T-cells in the periphery. If negative, a daily therapeutic dose of the medication is given at home for 4 to 5 days. These challenges would be contraindicated in severe drug reactions (DRESS, SJS/TEN).

Testing in the Primary Care Clinic and When to Refer to Allergy

Not all drug reactions need to be referred to an allergist, and in fact, most penicillin allergies may be safely performed in a primary care office. First, many adverse effects are incorrectly labeled as an allergy. For expected side effects such as gastrointestinal symptoms, headache, and noncutaneous reactions, these can be delabeled as an allergy without the need for further testing. Side effects can be managed symptomatically if the patient needed penicillin.

In cases of mild delayed rashes (Type IVa reactions), the graded challenge, as described above, is safe and can be performed by primary care doctors. In many cases, penicillin allergy may be cleared by challenges without the need for skin testing or patch testing.

Referral to an allergist can be considered in several scenarios. Reactions that were recent (within past 5 years) and those associated with Type I/IgE symptoms (hives/angioedema, respiratory symptoms, cardiovascular symptoms) should be referred for skin testing. Reactions that involved drug-induced hemolysis or any other cytopenia are considered severe and should be referred for further workup. Furthermore, any drug allergy reaction that produced fever, elevated blood eosinophils, oral (or other mucosal surface) lesions, elevated liver enzymes or altered renal function, or blistering rashes would be considered moderate-to-severe and would warrant referral.

SUMMARY

Allergy to penicillin can occur via any of the 4 types of Gel-Coombs hypersensitivity reactions, producing distinct clinical histories and physical examination findings. These range in severity from mild reactions where the culprit drug may be used again, to severe reactions that necessitate lifelong avoidance. For all drug reactions, immediate penicillin discontinuation is essential, and depending on the type of reaction, epinephrine, antihistamines, and/or glucocorticoids may be used. Most beta-lactams may be safely used in penicillin-allergic patients, with the possible exception of first-generation and second-generation cephalosporins. It is important to note that most patients lose Type I and Type IVa allergies over time, so testing can be extremely useful in these reactions. Penicillin testing includes skin testing, patch testing, and graded challenge. The selection of the type of testing depends on the clinical setting, equipment availability, and type of hypersensitivity reaction. Desensitization may be used in some cases where treatment with penicillins is essential.

CLINICS CARE POINTS

- History and physical exam are essential to characterize the type of hypersensitivity reaction.
- During an acute reaction, prompt discontinuation of penicillin and appropriate treatment are essential.
- Anaphylaxis should be treated with epinephrine.
- Prednisone is the mainstay of treatment of Type IVb reactions (DRESS).
- Type IVc reactions (SJS/TEN) require supportive care and possible transfer to a burn center.
- Type IVa reactions are often mild and penicillins may be used again if needed.
- Most patients lose Type I-meditated and Type IVa-mediated hypersensitivities to penicillin during a 5 to 10-year period.
- Penicillin skin testing and/or graded challenges can be helpful to determine whether the allergy has been lost.

DISCLOSURE

None of the authors has a financial or commercial conflict of interest. None of the authors has any funding.

REFERENCES

1. Castells M, Khan DA, Phillips EJ. Penicillin allergy. N Engl J Med 2019;381(24): 2338–51.
2. Bernstein L, Bloomberg G, Castells M, et al. Drug allergy: an updated practice parameter. Ann Allergy Asthma Immunol 2010;105(4):259–73.e78.
3. Macy E, Shu Y-H. The effect of penicillin allergy testing on future health care utilization: a matched cohort study. J Allergy Clin Immunol Pract 2017;5(3):705–10.

4. Baman N, VanNostrand B, Ishmael F. Prevalence of penicillin allergy and adverse outcomes in geriatric inpatients at a tertiary care hospital. J Allergy Clin Immunol 2012;129(2):AB102.

5. Reddy V, Baman NS, Whitener C, et al. Drug resistant infections with methicillin-resistant staphylococcus aureus, clostridium difficile, and vancomycin resistant enterococcus are associated with a higher prevalence of penicillin allergy. J Allergy Clin Immunol 2013;131(2):AB170.

6. Reddy V, Ishmael FT. Vancomycin use and vancomycin resistant enterococcus are increased in patients with reported penicillin allergy. J Allergy Clin Immunol 2014;133(2):AB271.

7. Macy E, Contreras R. Health care use and serious infection prevalence associated with penicillin "allergy" in hospitalized patients: a cohort study. J Allergy Clin Immunol 2014;133(3):790–6.

8. Sousa-Pinto B, Blumenthal KG, Macy E, et al. Penicillin allergy testing is cost-saving: an economic evaluation study. Clin Infect Dis Off Publ Infect Dis Soc Am 2020;72(6):924–38.

9. Parser CW, deWeck AL, Kern M, et al. The preparation and some properties of penicillenic acid derivatives relevant to penicillin hypersensitivity. J Exp Med 1962;115(4):803–19.

10. Ishmael FT, Panganiban RP, Zhang S. Drug allergy and adverse drug reactions. In: Craig T, Ledford DK, editors. Allergy and asthma. Cham: Springer International Publishing; 2018. p. 1–14.

11. Levine BB, Ovary Z. Studies on the mechanism of the formation of the penicillin antigen. J Exp Med 1961;114(6):875–940.

12. Picard M, Paradis L, Bégin P, et al. Skin testing only with penicillin g in children with a history of penicillin allergy. Ann Allergy Asthma Immunol 2014;113(1): 75–81.

13. Blanca M, Torres MJ, García JJ, et al. Natural evolution of skin test sensitivity in patients allergic to β-lactam antibiotics. J Allergy Clin Immunol 1999;103(5): 918–24.

14. Sullivan TJ, Wedner HJ, Shatz GS, et al. Skin testing to detect penicillin allergy. J Allergy Clin Immunol 1981;68(3):171–80.

15. Aster RH, Curtis BR, McFARLAND JG, et al. Drug-induced immune thrombocytopenia: pathogenesis, diagnosis, and management. J Thromb Haemost 2009;7(6): 911–8.

16. George JN, Aster RH. Drug-induced thrombocytopenia: pathogenesis, evaluation, and management. Hematology 2009;2009(1):153–8.

17. Blumenthal KG, Peter JG, Trubiano JA, et al. Antibiotic allergy. Lancet 2019; 393(10167):183–98.

18. Demoly P, Adkinson NF, Brockow K, et al. International consensus on drug allergy. Allergy 2014;69(4):420–37.

19. Pichler WJ, Adam J, Watkins S, et al. Drug hypersensitivity: how drugs stimulate t cells via pharmacological interaction with immune receptors. Int Arch Allergy Immunol 2015;168(1):13–24.

20. Vocanson M, Hennino A, Rozières A, et al. Effector and regulatory mechanisms in allergic contact dermatitis: pathophysiology of contact dermatitis. Allergy 2009; 64(12):1699–714.

21. Bechara R, Feray A, Pallardy M. Drug and chemical allergy: a role for a specific naive t-cell repertoire? Front Immunol 2021;12:653102.

22. Mill C, Primeau M-N, Medoff E, et al. Assessing the diagnostic properties of a graded oral provocation challenge for the diagnosis of immediate and nonimmediate reactions to amoxicillin in children. JAMA Pediatr 2016;170(6):e160033.
23. Musette P, Janela B. New insights into drug reaction with eosinophilia and systemic symptoms pathophysiology. Front Med 2017;4:179.
24. Kano Y, Ishida T, Hirahara K, et al. Visceral involvements and long-term sequelae in drug-induced hypersensitivity syndrome. Med Clin North Am 2010;94(4):743–59.
25. Cacoub P, Musette P, Descamps V, et al. The DRESS syndrome: a literature review. Am J Med 2011;124(7):588–97.
26. Lerch M, Mainetti C, Terziroli Beretta-Piccoli B, et al. Current perspectives on stevens-johnson syndrome and toxic epidermal necrolysis. Clin Rev Allergy Immunol 2018;54(1):147–76.
27. Schneider JA, Cohen PR. Stevens-johnson syndrome and toxic epidermal necrolysis: a concise review with a comprehensive summary of therapeutic interventions emphasizing supportive measures. Adv Ther 2017;34(6):1235–44.
28. Sekula P, Dunant A, Mockenhaupt M, et al. Comprehensive survival analysis of a cohort of patients with stevens–johnson syndrome and toxic epidermal necrolysis. J Invest Dermatol 2013;133(5):1197–204.
29. Britschgi M, Greyerz S, Burkhart C, et al. Molecular aspects of drug recognition by specific T cells. Curr Drug Targets 2003;4(1):1–11.
30. Tokura Y, Mori T, Hino R. Psoriasis and other Th17-mediated skin diseases. J UOEH 2010;32(4):317–28.
31. Szatkowski J, Schwartz RA. Acute generalized exanthematous pustulosis (AGEP): a review and update. J Am Acad Dermatol 2015;73(5):843–8.
32. Lieberman P, Kemp S, Oppenheimer J, et al. The diagnosis and management of anaphylaxis: an updated practice parameter. J Allergy Clin Immunol 2005;115(3):S483–523.
33. Sampson HA, Muñoz-Furlong A, Campbell RL, et al. Second symposium on the definition and management of anaphylaxis: summary report—second national institute of allergy and infectious disease/food allergy and anaphylaxis network symposium. Ann Emerg Med 2006;47(4):373–80.
34. Kaliner M, Austen KF. Cyclic AMP, ATP, and reversed anaphylactic histamine release from rat mast cells. J Immunol 1974;112(2):664–74.
35. Simons KJ, Simons FER. Epinephrine and its use in anaphylaxis: current issues. Curr Opin Allergy Clin Immunol 2010;10(4):354–61.
36. Simons FER, Ardusso LRF, Bilò MB, et al. World allergy organization anaphylaxis guidelines: summary. J Allergy Clin Immunol 2011;127(3):587–93.e22.
37. Shaker M, Toy D, Lindholm C, et al. Summary and simulation of reported adverse events from epinephrine autoinjectors and a review of the literature. J Allergy Clin Immunol Pract 2018;6(6):2143–5.e4.
38. Nurmatov UB, Rhatigan E, Simons FER, et al. H2-Antihistamines for the treatment of anaphylaxis with and without shock: a systematic review. Ann Allergy Asthma Immunol 2014;112(2):126–31.
39. Michelson KA, Monuteaux MC, Neuman MI. Glucocorticoids and hospital length of stay for children with anaphylaxis: a retrospective study. J Pediatr 2015;167(3):719–24.e3.
40. Liyanage C, Galappatthy P, Seneviratne S. Corticosteroids in managment of anaphylaxis: a systematic review of evidence. Eur Annu Allergy Clin Immunol 2017;49(5):196–207.

41. Garratty G. Drug-induced immune hemolytic anemia. Hematol Am Soceity Hematol Educ Program 2009;73–9. https://doi.org/10.1182/asheducation-2009.1.73.
42. Mayer B, Bartolmäs T, Yürek S, et al. Variability of findings in drug-induced immune haemolytic anaemia: experience over 20 years in a single centre. Transfus Med Hemotherapy 2015;42(5):333–9.
43. Hill QA, Stamps R, Massey E, et al. The British Society for Haematology Guidelines. Guidelines on the management of drug-induced immune and secondary autoimmune, haemolytic anaemia. Br J Haematol 2017;177(2):208–20.
44. Leicht, H. B.; Weinig, E.; Mayer, B., et al Ceftriaxone-induced hemolytic anemia with severe renal failure: a case report and review of literature. BMC Pharmacol Toxicol 2018, 19 (1), 67. .
45. Garratty G. Immune hemolytic anemia associated with drug therapy. Blood Rev 2010;24(4–5):143–50.
46. Pierce A, Nester T. Pathology Consultation on drug-induced hemolytic anemia. Am J Clin Pathol 2011;136(1):7–12.
47. Karunathilaka, H. G. C. S.; Chandrasiri, D. P.; Ranasinghe, P., et al Co-Amoxiclav induced immune haemolytic anaemia: a case report. Case Rep Hematol 2020, 2020, 1–3. .
48. Tatum, A. J.; Ditto, A. M.; Patterson, R. Severe serum sickness-like reaction to oral penicillin drugs: three case reports. Ann Allergy Asthma Immunol 2001, 86 (3), 330–334. .
49. Shiohara T, Mizukawa Y. Drug-induced hypersensitivity syndrome (DiHS)/drug reaction with eosinophilia and systemic symptoms (DRESS): an update in 2019. Allergol Int 2019;68(3):301–8.
50. Shiga S, Cartotto R. What are the fluid requirements in toxic epidermal necrolysis? J Burn Care Res 2010;31(1):100–4.
51. Coss-Bu JA, Jefferson LS, Levy ML, et al. Nutrition requirements in patients with toxic epidermal necrolysis. Nutr Clin Pract 1997;12(2):81–4.
52. Valeyrie-Allanore L, Ingen-Housz-Oro S, Chosidow O, et al. French referral center managment of stevens-johnson syndrome/toxic epidermal necrolysis. Dermatol Sin 2013;31(4):191–5.
53. de Prost N, Ingen-Housz-Oro S, Duong T anh, et al. Bacteremia in stevens-johnson syndrome and toxic epidermal necrolysis: epidemiology, risk factors, and predictive value of skin cultures. Medicine (Baltimore) 2010;89(1):28–36.
54. Hasegawa A, Abe R. Recent advances in managing and understanding stevens-johnson syndrome and toxic epidermal necrolysis. F1000Research 2020;9:612.
55. French LE. Toxic epidermal necrolysis and stevens johnson syndrome: our current understanding. Allergol Int 2006;55(1):9–16.
56. Feldmeyer L, Heidemeyer K, Yawalkar N. Acute generalized exanthematous pustulosis: pathogenesis, genetic background, clinical variants and therapy. Int J Mol Sci 2016;17(8):1214.
57. Davidovici BB, Pavel D, Cagnano E, et al. Acute generalized exanthematous pustulosis following a spider bite: report of 3 cases. J Am Acad Dermatol 2006;55(3): 525–9.
58. Buettiker U, Keller M, Pichler WJ, et al. Oral prednisolone induced acute generalized exanthematous pustulosis due to corticosteroids of group a confirmed by epicutaneous testing and lymphocyte transformation tests. Dermatology 2006; 213(1):40–3.
59. Chang S, Huang Y, Yang C, et al. Clinical manifestations and characteristics of patients with acute generalized exanthematous pustulosis in Asia. Acta Derm Venereol 2008;88(4):363–5.

60. Pumphery RSH, Davis S. Under-reporting of antibiotic anaphylaxis may put patients at risk. The Lancet 1999;353(9159):1157–8.
61. St NB. Drug allergy: an updated practice parameter. Ann Allergy 2010;105:78.
62. Romano A, Viola M, Guéant-Rodriguez R-M, et al. Imipenem in patients with immediate hypersensitivity to penicillins. N Engl J Med 2006;354(26):2835–7.
63. Sogn D, Evans R III, Sheperd G, et al. Results of the national institute of allergy and infectious diseases collaborative clinical trial to test the predictive value of skin testing with major and minor penicillin derivatives in hospitalized adults. Arch Intern Med 1992;152(5):1025–32.
64. Gadde J, Spence M, Wheeler B, et al. Clinical experience with penicillin skin testing in a large inner-city STD clinic. JAMA 1993;270(20):2456–63.
65. Solley G, Gleich G, Vandellen R. Penicillin allergy: clinical experience with a battery of skin-test reagents. J Allergy Clin Immunol 1982;69(2):238–44.
66. Green G, Rosenblum A, Sweet L. Evaluation of penicillin hypersensitivity: value of clinical history and skin testing with penicilloyl-polylysine and penicillin G A cooperative prospective study of the penicillin study group of the american academy of allergy. J Allergy Clin Immunol 1977;60(6):339–45.
67. Broyles AD, Banerji A, Barmettler S, et al. Practical guidance for the evaluation and management of drug hypersensitivity: specific drugs. J Allergy Clin Immunol Pract 2020;8(9):S16–116.
68. Romano A, Blanca M, Torres MJ, et al. EAACI interest group on drug hypersensitivity. Diagnosis of Nonimmediate Reactions to Beta-Lactam Antibiotics. Allergy 2004;59(11):1153–60.
69. Padial A, Antunez C, Blanca-Lopez N, et al. Non-immediate reactions to β-lactams: diagnostic value of skin testing and drug provocation test. Clin Exp Allergy 2008;38(5):822–8.

Urticaria and Angioedema

Kate Szymanski, DO*, Paul Schaefer, MD, PhD

KEYWORDS

- Acute urticaria • Chronic urticaria • Angioedema • Antihistamines

KEY POINTS

- Urticaria is a rash of well-circumscribed, pruritic raised wheals and can be the first symptom of a severe allergic reaction.
- Angioedema presents as localized non-pitting edema in the face or extremities that may be warm and painful, with or without urticaria.
- Urticaria and angioedema are caused by immunoglobulin E- and non-immunoglobulin E-mediated release of histamine and other inflammatory mediators primarily from mast cells.
- Initial treatment includes avoidance of triggers (for acute urticaria) and second-generation antihistamines.
- Urticaria can be acute or chronic.

INTRODUCTION: URTICARIA AND ANGIOEDEMA

Urticaria, commonly called hives, is a dermatologic condition that presents with very pruritic, well-circumscribed, raised wheals ranging from several millimeters to several centimeters or larger in size.[1] Individual wheals develop rapidly over minutes and may change shape or coalesce, forming rings, serpiginous or map-like patterns, or giant wheals.[2] Individual wheals typically last for a few hours and should resolve within 24 hours, though new crops can recur repeatedly. They can be pale to erythematous and blanch under pressure.[3] Angioedema is localized, non-pitting edema, often warm and painful. It occurs primarily on the face and extremities. Urticaria and angioedema can occur separately or concomitantly.

Urticaria and angioedema are commonly seen in the primary care setting.[4] Urticaria has a lifetime prevalence of about 10% to 20%. Higher risk populations include children, middle-aged women, and individuals with a history of allergies. The associated intense pruritus can cause significant impairment in daily functioning[1] and disrupt sleep. Although often self-limited and benign, urticaria and angioedema can be symptoms of life-threatening anaphylaxis or is rarely associated with significant underlying disease. Angioedema that impedes the upper airway can be life-threatening.

Department of Family Medicine, College of Medicine and Life Sciences at the University of Toledo Medical Center, 3333 Glendale Avenue, Toledo, OH 43614-2598, USA
* Corresponding author. 3333 Glendale Avenue, Toledo, OH 43614.
E-mail address: kate.szymanski@utoledo.edu

Prim Care Clin Office Pract 50 (2023) 237–252
https://doi.org/10.1016/j.pop.2022.11.003
0095-4543/23/© 2022 Elsevier Inc. All rights reserved.

Definitions

Urticaria can be acute or chronic. Urticaria occurring for less than 6 weeks is termed acute urticaria. Urticaria occurring for most days for 6 weeks or more is called chronic urticaria. Urticaria can also be classified as spontaneous, where there is no clear trigger, and inducible where a noted stimulus elicits symptoms.

DISCUSSION: ACUTE URTICARIA
Pathogenesis

The primary cell involvement with urticaria is the mast cells present in the dermis and subdermis. Activated mast cells produce pro-inflammatory and vasodilatory substances. The release of these substances in the superficial dermis causes urticaria, whereas such release in the deeper dermis or subdermis causes angioedema (see below). In the acute phase, these chemicals are responsible for pruritus, swelling, and erythema. Acute phase substances include histamine, leukotrienes C4, and prostaglandin D2. Bradykinin release causes increased vascular permeability, therefore increasing the local edema and influx of inflammatory cells.[5] In the delayed phase of an urticarial reaction, there is also secretion of inflammatory cytokines including tumor necrosis factor (TNF)-alpha, interleukin (IL)-4, and IL-5.[6] These delayed phase inflammatory cytokines cause an influx of inflammatory cells to the affected area leading to additional edema, erythema, and pruritus. Urticarial lesions can be seen in **Fig. 1** with an urticarial ring on the lateral shoulder and **Fig. 2** with a diffuse urticarial reaction which was interfering with sleep.

Causes

There are a number of potential triggers of acute urticaria (**Table 1**). The history and physical examination should seek to identify possible causes.

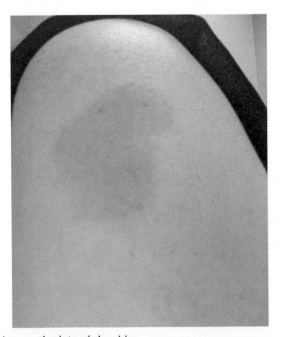

Fig. 1. Urticarial ring on the lateral shoulder.

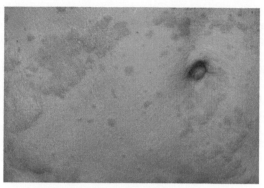

Fig. 2. Diffuse urticarial reaction which was interfering with sleep.

In cases of a singular event of hives, the urticaria could be secondary to an infection which will self-resolve within days to weeks. Commonly, infective urticaria is from a virus such as common upper respiratory viruses. Viral hepatitides and HIV are also associated with urticaria, but these are rare causes of urticaria. In children, the most common cause of urticaria is infection.

Another common cause of acute urticaria is a drug reaction or allergy. In this instance, symptoms typically start within minutes up to hours after the medication exposure. Common medications causing allergic acute urticaria include antibiotics such as beta lactams, radiocontrast media, sedatives, and sulfonamides.[7] Medications such as nonsteroidal anti-inflammatories and opioids can trigger mast cell release directly, as can ethyl alcohol.

Alternatively, food allergies can result in acute urticaria or angioedema.[8] The urticarial reaction may be perioral which is diagnostically challenging to differentiate from early angioedema. Common food allergens include milk, eggs, peanuts, tree nuts, shellfish, finned fish, wheat, sesame, and soy. Food pseudoallergens are foods or

Table 1
Causes of urticaria and angioedema

Cause	Notes
Allergens	Contact, food, airborne, insect venom
Autoimmune disease	Various connective tissue disorders
Cryoglobulinemia	Hepatitis C, lymphoma, leukemia
Food pseudoallergens	Foods and food additives containing histamine or histamine releasing compounds
Infections	Viral, bacterial, parasitic, fungal
Mastocytosis	Pathological accumulation of mast cells in skin and other tissues
Medications	Allergic reactions, direct mast cell degranulation, bradykinin increase
Neoplasm	Lymphoma, leukemia, myeloma, germ cell tumors
Physical/environmental stimuli	Dermatographism, cold, heat, pressure, vibration, sunlight (uncommon), water (rare)
Vasculitis	Immune complex deposition

Data from Refs.[5,20,21]

food additives, including food coloring, which have small amounts of histamine or directly trigger the release of histamine causing an allergic reaction via a different mechanism.[5] Reactions due to food allergy can lead to anaphylaxis, and patients must always carry epinephrine with them.

Approximately 30% of patients with an acute urticarial event will have intermittent recurrent episodes that do not meet diagnostic criteria for chronic urticaria. Some cases of repeated acute urticaria are noticeably secondary to exposure to an allergen or other trigger and will occur within hours of exposure. Allergic patients are often aware of their allergen(s) and will be able to identify the cause when asked by the clinician. When unclear etiology is present with recurrent urticarial attacks, evaluation for nonallergic causes including hepatitis, thyroid disease, and leukemia may be warranted.

Diagnosis

Urticaria is a clinical diagnosis based on history and physical examination. Patients should be asked about possible exposures such as chemicals, food, medications (including supplements), and contact with animals, plants, or metals for acute urticaria. More definitive diagnosis can be elicited when exposure history is combined with history of timing of lesions, localization and distribution of urticaria, and systemic complaints.[9] Known allergies, travel history, family history of similar symptoms, and history of recent infectious exposure should be explored. A sexual history and illicit drug use history may shed light on the risk of viral hepatitides and HIV infection. A thorough review of systems can help identify the presence of underlying systemic disease. Physical examination should include vitals and skin examination, including characterization of lesions and the presence or absence of dermatographism, along with cardiovascular and pulmonary examination. Other elements of underlying disease to look for include examination for hepatomegaly, lymphadenopathy, synovitis, and thyromegaly. If individual wheals have been persistent for greater than 24 hours, a skin biopsy is recommended. Urticaria is commonly seen in multiple clinical settings, and providers should be comfortable and confident with their examination skills regarding this diagnosis.

Current guidelines do not recommend laboratory workup for acute urticaria in the absence of concerning symptoms such as hives lasting longer than 48 hours, scarring, or bruising on resolution. For chronic urticaria, workup may include complete blood count (CBC) with diff, erythrocyte sedimentation rate (ESR)/CRP, thyroid stimulating hormone (TSH), and liver function test (LFTs). For both acute and chronic urticaria, additional focused laboratory tests should be done only when the history or physical examination suggests underlying causes or systemic disease.

Allergy testing is not recommended unless history suggests an allergic cause. Immunoglobulin E (IgE) food panel testing should not be completed as part of the initial workup.[8] Skin testing is used in diagnosing the etiology of acute urticaria with foods, insect venom, and medications. Although allergy testing may be beneficial for advanced treatment modalities, the initial diagnosis is not dependent on this testing. Intradermal skin testing and IgE testing for food allergies has a high false-positive rate.[8] Strong clinical correlation is recommended with positive food skin testing given the high false-positive rate and can be confirmed with a monitored oral food challenge in the appropriate setting. Appropriate testing in the setting of a supportive clinical history can increase your posttest probability of a true positive.

Differential

There are several medical conditions as shown in **Table 2**, which can cause pruritic rashes that can mimic the symptomatology of urticaria. Many of these can be excluded based on the history of presenting illness and physical examination. Some

Table 2
Differential diagnoses for urticaria

Condition	Notes
Allergic dermatitis	Maculopapular or vesicular lesions, longer duration, erythema, distribution consistent with exposure, may have scaling
Drug eruption/exanthem	Maculopapular to bullous, medication history
Erythema multiforme	Target lesions, longer duration, fever
Henoch–Schonlein purpura (IgA vasculitis)	Purpuric lesions on lower extremities, abdominal pain, arthralgias
Insect bite	Punctum may be identifiable, exposure history
Mastocytosis	Yellow/orange/brown color, Darier's sign (wheal and flare from stroking lesion)
Pityriasis rosea	Herald patch, lesions oriented along skin fold lines (Christmas tree pattern), lesions persist for weeks
Psoriasis	Distribution of lesions, non-blanching, scaling
Pruritic urticarial papules and plaques of pregnancy	Third trimester of pregnancy, lesions primarily on abdomen
Scabies	Papular, characteristic distribution, burrows may be detectable
Stevens–Johnson syndrome	Prodrome, macular to bullae, pain, mucosal involvement, Nikolsky sign
Viral exanthem-varicella, measles, mumps, rubella	Viral prodrome, characteristic lesions

Data from Refs.[5,20–22]

more serious illnesses that should be recognized quickly and treated appropriately would include Henoch–Schönlein purpura, erythema multiforme, and Stevens–Johnson syndrome.

One illness which can mimic symptomatology of acute urticaria is new psoriasis which would be easily differentiated by lack of blanching and significant scale. Alternatively, contact dermatitis can often be confounded with urticaria but will often present in a distribution consistent with the area of contact, which may be diagnostic. Another common reaction is a drug eruption or exanthem such as the reaction that can be seen when patients suffering from mononucleosis receive amoxicillin. Pityriasis rosea has a herald patch which is erythematous and pruritic but shortly followed by the eruption of a Christmas tree pattern rash across the trunk.

The viral exanthem for varicella helps differentiate it from urticarial vasculitis in most cases, but if needed, biopsy can differentiate these illnesses. Measles and mumps have a very classic viral exanthem which is distinguishable due to the lack of pruritus and classical history of viral illness. Fortunately, these illnesses are seen less often due to vaccination. A common infection with scabies should be easily differentiated based on the location and history of contact with infected source.

Treatment

Sudden rash can be one of the first symptoms of a severe allergic reaction called anaphylaxis. Anaphylaxis must be ruled out in all cases of acute urticaria by assessing airway patency, respiratory status, blood pressure, and abdominal symptoms. After potential severe illness has been ruled out, conservative treatment can be started. The mainstay of treatment of acute urticaria is avoidance of triggers and antihistamine therapy as needed. For some patients, topical antihistamines may be sufficient, but often oral antihistamines are required and there can be concern for rebound with topicals. The most well-tolerated initial treatment regimen would be a second-generation antihistamine such as cetirizine, desloratadine, fexofenadine, levocetirizine, or loratadine, which can be titrated higher than normal dose regimens. We recommend starting with the standard dosage of the second-generation antihistamine of choice. If symptoms are not controlled this can be sequentially increased to double and then quadruple the standard dose. Common reasons that antihistamines are not effective would include insufficient strength, low-dose, or insufficient treatment period.[10] Given that these medications are often given at higher dose than otherwise recommended, there is an increased risk of side effects and doses and drug interactions should be noted and monitored.[11] Non-steroidal anti-inflammatory drug (NSAIDs) and alcohol should be avoided.

If second-generation antihistamines are insufficient at doses two to four times the standard dose, changing second-generation antihistamine or addition of a second agent may be required (see chronic urticaria: treatment below). First-generation antihistamines such as diphenhydramine and hydroxyzine may be added at night as symptoms are often more disruptive to sleep. In addition, there are parenteral formulations, which can be useful in urgent or emergent care settings. Patients should have close follow-up with their primary care provider for follow-up of symptom management and ongoing evaluation for changes in illness.

SUMMARY

Acute urticaria is less than 6 weeks of a pruritic urticarial rash and can be the first symptom of a severe allergic reaction. Onset can be very rapid, and symptoms can last hours to days. Causes are diverse and include medications, food, viruses, and contact irritants. The diagnosis is made clinically, and treatment should be initiated early with second-generation antihistamines that can be titrated to two to four times the standard dose.

DISCUSSION: CHRONIC URTICARIA
Diagnosis

The prevalence of chronic urticaria is less than 1% of the general population. Chronic urticaria may be spontaneous, inducible, autoimmune, vasculitic, pseudoallergenic, infectious or idiopathic.[12] Morphology, distribution, history, and timeline may help differentiate the underlying etiology of the urticaria.[11] In chronic urticaria, a trigger or clear cause may be identified in only 10% to 20% of cases. There is a 2:1 female-to-male ratio and disease onset is most prominent in the third to fifth decades of life. This is generally a self-limited condition with an average duration of 1 to 5 years, though it can be very challenging for patients and clinicians.[10]

Pathogenesis

Chronic idiopathic urticaria currently has an unclear pathophysiology. Some cases of chronic urticaria are believed to have immunogenic stimuli, which may involve the complement cascade including C3a and C5a augmentation of histamine release.[11] Many cases of chronic urticaria remain unexplained despite well-known auto antibodies against IgE or the high-affinity IgE receptor in approximately 30% to 50% of chronic patients.[12] Some studies suggest an autologous skin reaction with activation of basophils causing functional autoantibodies. This is still under investigation as some studies also suggest this autologous skin reaction can be found in otherwise healthy subjects.[6] In contrast to acute urticaria, some investigations have demonstrated upregulation of TNF-alpha in patients with chronic idiopathic urticaria.[12]

Subclassification

Chronic urticaria is subdivided based on the reported underlying etiology. Subdivisions include physical factors, idiopathic, autoimmune, vasculitic, pseudoallergenic, and infectious.[12] Physical urticaria accounts for 15% to 30% of all chronic urticaria cases.[4,12] Approximately 75% to 85% of cases of chronic urticaria are diagnosed as idiopathic.[4,6] Infective and vasculitis urticarial rashes are typically longer lasting and should be ruled out if any red flag symptoms are present.

Chronic inducible urticaria

Urticaria due to physical stimuli is also called chronic inducible urticaria. This is a subtype of urticaria that may require patients to alter their lifestyle in order to avoid urticaria-triggering stimuli and is less likely to spontaneously resolve. Urticaria can be triggered by physical stimuli such as sunlight, pressure, cold, heat, vibration, or rarely water. Physical urticaria can occur in individuals that have other forms of hives as well.[7] Once a physical factor has been identified this should be avoided as much as is feasible.[9]

Cholinergic urticaria is sometimes known as generalized heat urticaria in which increased body temperature, including with exercise, triggers diffuse hives. Heat is a common trigger for many people, which can be challenging to avoid and items such as tight clothing or rubber bands may exacerbate their symptoms. Typically, this diagnosis is made based on history and physical alone, but if confirmation is required exposure to heat in the office can be diagnostic.[3]

If hives develop from scratching or from rubbing of the skin, it is called dermatographism. Dermatographism is the most common of the physical urticaria affecting approximately 5% of all patients with urticaria and up to 30% of patients with physical urticaria. This form of urticaria is easily reproduced in the office with the use of a firm blunt object on the patient's skin triggering linear symptomatic urticarial lesions. In **Fig. 3**, the urticarial reaction after moving a necklace during appointment. The

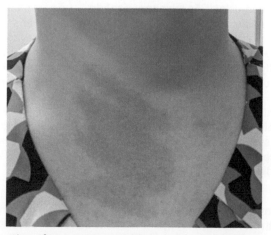

Fig. 3. Urticarial reaction after moving a necklace during appointment.

response may be blunted if the patient is using antihistamines. It is important to note that this form of urticaria does not involve the mucosal tissue or trigger angioedema.[11]

An important form of chronic inducible urticaria is secondary to cold stimuli. Symptoms typically occur when exposed to cold such as standing in front of an air conditioner, holding cold objects, or while in the freezer section of the grocery store. The diagnosis is based on history and the ice cube test. This test entails placing a frozen object, such as an ice cube (typically in a plastic bag), on the patient's forearm for 4 minutes after which a large hive mimicking the shape of the frozen object will form. Most of the cases are idiopathic, but underlying etiologies must be evaluated including cold agglutinin, paroxysmal cold hemoglobinuria, cryoglobulinemia, and cryofibrinogenemia.[11] It is very important that these patients are counseled never to swim alone as total body exposure can result in hypotension from significant mediator release.[7]

Idiopathic

Chronic idiopathic urticaria is defined by episodes of short-lived recurrent pruritic wheals without a defined underlying etiology. This is a diagnosis of exclusion, and biopsy is often involved. The duration of disease burden is variable with an average of 3 to 5 years. Auto antibodies are believed to be an underlying cause, and autoimmune disease should be ruled out including Hashimoto's thyroiditis, as antithyroid antibodies occur between 15% and 24% of the time in idiopathic urticaria.[7] Other causes that should be ruled out include medication-induced, contact irritant, and chronic illness.[12] Systemic chronic illnesses such as mastocytosis, Hashimoto's thyroiditis, Sjogren's syndrome, rheumatoid arthritis, lymphoma, systemic lupus erythematosus, celiac disease, and chronic hepatitis B or C should be ruled out in chronic idiopathic urticaria if there is suspicion based on findings.[3]

Autoimmune

The clinical presentation of patients with autoimmune urticaria is similar to nonautoimmune-based disease. The autoimmune basis for urticaria was initially observed in 1983 by Leznoff and colleagues[13] after observation of the association between chronic idiopathic urticaria and thyroid disease. Testing with autologous serum skin tests and high-affinity IgE receptors has found that there is a substantial histamine released activity independent of cell bound IgE suggesting the presence of functional autoantibodies against the high-affinity IgE receptor on mast cells and basophils. In addition, the role of complement in the autoantibody-mediated histamine release cannot be reproduced using C5a inhibitory peptide.

To date, the gold standard for diagnosing autoimmune urticaria with functional autoantibodies is a basophil histamine release assay. This bioassay requires fresh basophils from healthy donors making it difficult to standardize and likely confined to research. Currently, the best in vivo clinical test is autologous skin serum testing with a sensitivity of approximately 70% and specificity of 80%, typically performed by a specialist.[11]

Autoimmune urticaria has also been associated with several diseases such as neoplasms, rheumatoid arthritis, autoimmune thyroid disease, systemic lupus erythematosus, Schnitzler syndrome, and Muckle–Wells syndrome. Although treatment of an underlying disease can be beneficial, symptomatic therapy is the same as with other chronic urticaria disease processes.[12]

Vasculitic

This is a form of small vessel vasculitis that may be present in urticaria or autoimmune diseases. This rash can be seen in **Figs. 4** and **5**, which show a bilateral lower extremity, biopsy proven, case of vasculitic urticaria due to a drug reaction. Atypical lesions

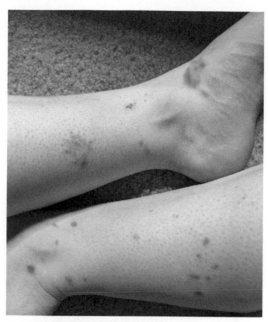

Fig. 4. Lesions of urticarial vasculitis.

such as those that do not blanch, leave behind pigment changes following resolution, or last longer than 24 hours are associated with urticarial vasculitis.[3] This urticarial rash can have small vessels which is confounding to the diagnosis as shown in **Fig. 6**. This form of urticaria may be associated with injury to the small vessels of organs such as kidney, eye, lung, or central nervous system. It is very important to diagnose this early and treated aggressively due to the risk of significant morbidity and underlying serious illness and sequelae.[14] Common systemic diseases include systemic lupus erythematosus, Sjogren's syndrome, Lyme disease, infectious mononucleosis, Epstein–Barr virus, or hepatitis.[11]

Etiology is believed to be secondary to immune complexes in small blood vessels activating the complement system and mast cell degranulation. Diagnosis must be confirmed by skin biopsy which will reveal endothelial cell damage leukocytoclastic vasculitis and fibrin deposition with deposition of IgG and complement on immunofluorescence staining.[7]

Pseudoallergenic

Pseudoallergic reactions are a food or chemical triggering an allergic-mimicking reaction. Pseudoallergic urticaria typically presents 4 to 6 hours after the ingestion of the inciting substance. These reactions are usually not life-threatening and can be persistent through life. Common pseudoallergens include artificial food dyes, preservatives, sweeteners, and volatile aromatic compounds. This is very common in infants and children. Symptoms are usually not reproducible on provocation testing.[15] Foods which trigger pseudoallergic reactions are thought to have small amounts of histamine or directly cause the release of histamine, thereby triggering an allergic reaction.[5] There has been some discussion in the literature regarding hyperpermeability of the gastrointestinal track as a possible underlying etiology for pseudoallergic urticaria.[16] Avoidance of dietary pseudoallergens remains controversial in chronic urticaria, but

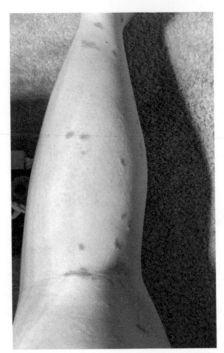

Fig. 5. Biopsy-proven vasculitic urticarial reactions of varying ages across the bilateral lower extremities.

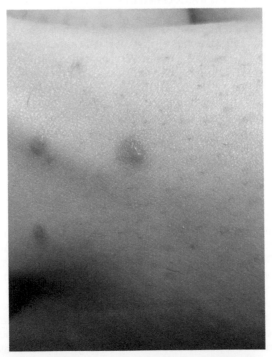

Fig. 6. Vasculitic vesicle with associated wheals as proven by biopsy.

for some patients in whom all other etiologies have been ruled out this may be beneficial. As with many dietary measures, compliance can be challenging.

Infection

Several infections are presumed to be affiliated with chronic urticaria. HIV infections have been associated with acute and chronic urticaria (notably cold-induced urticaria). Infection with *Helicobacter pylori* is controversial as a possible cause of chronic urticaria.[11] Although acute urticaria and urticarial vasculitis can be associated with upper respiratory tract infections, hepatitis, and infectious mononucleosis, there is insufficient evidence supporting a link with chronic urticaria.[7] Nonetheless, clinicians should treat noticeable infectious conditions even if affiliation to urticaria is unclear.[9] There is a possibility that a fungal infection such as onychomycosis and tinea pedis could elicit an urticarial reaction. There has been a reported association between parasitic infections such as strongyloidiasis, giardiasis, and amoebiasis.[17]

Differential

Chronic urticaria has much of the same differential as acute urticaria, with a few notable exceptions. Several of the common differential diagnoses were discussed in each subclassification for chronic urticaria. These include previously mentioned disorders including thyroid disease, Lyme disease, systemic lupus erythematosus, chronic hepatitis, rheumatoid arthritis, leukemia, celiac disease, and Sjogren's syndrome.[18] Although many of these conditions can be differentiated with skin biopsy, less invasive testing would include rheumatoid factor, thyroid function tests, IgE levels, hepatitis B and C screen, C-reactive protien (CRP)/ESR, and review of family history regarding hematologic cancers.

Treatment

Lesions can be distressing and interrupt normal daily function due to severe pruritus causing scratching with subsequent inflammation and irritant dermatitis. Nighttime symptoms can cause or worsen insomnia.[19] Although lesions are temporarily disfiguring, patient's perception of altered appearance can exacerbate underlying emotional stress exacerbating mental health illnesses. Treatment can be beneficial for both physical and emotional well-being.[3]

An algorithm for treating chronic urticaria is depicted in **Fig. 7**.[20,21] There are some differences between treatment guideline recommendations for chronic urticaria. The initial treatment of chronic urticaria in both guidelines is avoidance of identified triggers and use of second-generation antihistamines. In the American guidelines, the Joint Task Force on Practice Parameters,[20] if these agents fail to control symptoms in isolation, the next step in treatment can include titrating up to two to four times the normal dose of second-generation antihistamines or addition of one or more of several adjunctive therapies. Often 2 to 4 weeks is taken before stepping up therapy to appropriately determine response, though in severe cases or if a patient is at risk of airway involvement, these adjunctive therapies may be initiated at the start of treatment.[9] These adjunctive therapies include H_2 blockers such as cimetidine and famotidine, first-generation antihistamines, doxepin, and leukotriene receptor antagonists including montelukast and zafirlukast. If sleep is interrupted by pruritus the addition of a sedating first-generation antihistamine can be beneficial. Monotherapy with first-generation antihistamines is not ideal due to impairment of cognitive function due to sedating effect. Fortunately, most patients will become less affected by sedation with regular use of sedating antihistamines. Data on the efficacy of adjunctive treatment are modest. If patients remain unresponsive to antihistamine therapy with

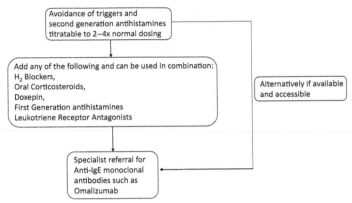

Fig. 7. Treatment algorithm for chronic urticaria. *See Refs.*[4,20,21]

adjunct therapy or if they have a flare of intense symptoms, a brief course of oral corticosteroids may be beneficial.[4] Referral to a specialist may be appropriate for additional treatment options. Anti-IgE monoclonal antibodies such as omalizumab have been shown to be highly efficacious for chronic urticaria and are the next step in treatment. Accessibility to specialty care and cost may be an issue for some patients. Alternative specialist therapy options include cyclosporine and hydroxychloroquine. Once control of symptoms has been established for 3 months, treatments can be stepwise titrated down and removed.

International guidelines[21] recommend initial treatment with second-generation antihistamines, titrated up to two to four times the normal dose. If this is insufficient, adjunctive therapies are not recommended, instead going directly to omalizumab given its proven efficacy.

SUMMARY

Chronic urticaria symptoms occur most days for greater than 6 weeks. The differential can be complex, and underlying illness should be ruled out. Initial treatment should include second-generation antihistamines, and all patients should avoid identified triggers. Anti-IgE monoclonal antibodies have been shown to be efficacious in chronic urticaria, and there are other potential adjunctive treatments. Consultation with a specialist may be appropriate.

DISCUSSION: ANGIOEDEMA

Angioedema is a sudden localized non-pitting swelling of the skin, subcutaneous tissues, or submucosa that typically resolves within 72 hours and is often recurrent.[7] The affected area is often warm and may be painful or burning. Mucosal surfaces are often involved. Angioedema commonly affects the eyes, lips, uvula, oropharynx, larynx, periorbital areas, genitals, hands, and feet. It can occur in other locations such as the bowel, where it can present as colicky abdominal pain, diarrhea, nausea, and vomiting. It can occur with or without urticaria. Angioedema can be a sign of anaphylaxis, which should be ruled out.

Pathogenesis

Angioedema is classically caused by mast cell degranulation or histaminergic causes as with urticaria (see above), and in such cases will typically present with urticaria and other signs of allergic reaction such as flushing. Angioedema can also be bradykinin-induced independent of mast cells; in such cases urticaria and itching are not present. Causes of bradykinin-induced angioedema include angiotensin-converting enzyme inhibitors (ACE inhibitors) and inherited or acquired C1 esterase inhibitor deficiencies. ACE inhibitors are the most common cause of bradykinin-induced angioedema.

Classification

Allergic
Allergic or histaminergic angioedema is caused by mast cell release of inflammatory compounds as described above for urticaria, but in the deeper dermis and subdermis. The approach to diagnosis is the same. It is often concurrent with urticaria. IgE-mediated food allergies often present as perioral, oral, and upper airway angioedema and can be life-threatening if they compromise the airway.

Angiotensin-converting enzyme inhibitors
ACE inhibitors can increase bradykinin levels resulting in increased vascular permeability and edema in susceptible areas. Less than 1 % of patients taking an ACE inhibitor will report angioedema, often perioral. It is more common in African Americans and women. This angioedema can present within weeks of starting the ACE inhibitor but may not present until after years of treatment. Episodes of angioedema can recur for up to months after stopping the medication. **Fig. 8** shows the angioedema of the lips from ACE inhibitors occurring several years after starting the medication.

C1 esterase inhibitor deficiencies
A deficiency in C1 esterase inhibitors can result in recurrent episodes of angioedema. Acquired C1 esterase inhibitor deficiencies can be associated with conditions such as malignancy and autoimmune disorders. Possible mechanisms include increased catabolism and autoantibodies. A rare cause is hereditary angioedema.

Idiopathic
As with chronic urticaria, in many cases, a cause of recurrent angioedema cannot be identified and are labeled idiopathic angioedema. Specialist referral may be appropriate.

DIAGNOSIS

The diagnosis of angioedema is likewise clinical based on a thorough history and physical examination. The approach is as described for urticaria, especially when urticaria is also present. Airway patency should be verified, and anaphylaxis ruled out. The absence of urticaria or other signs of allergic reaction should raise suspicion for bradykinin-induced angioedema. A review of medications is important, especially ACE inhibitors. Laboratory work for angioedema without urticaria can include

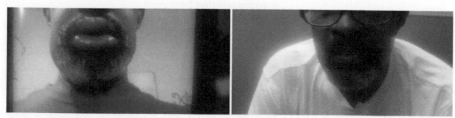

Fig. 8. Perioral angioedema due to an ACE inhibitor.

complement levels, especially C4. If C4 levels are low, C1 esterase inhibitor levels may be ordered. If bowel angioedema is suspected, abdominal ultrasound or CT may be helpful.

DIFFERENTIAL

Table 3 lists diagnoses that could be confused with angioedema. Lymphedema and myxedematous hypothyroidism cause non-pitting edema, though the time course on onset and resolution is much slower, as is in macroglossia from amyloidosis. Conditions that cause pitting edema, including liver failure, kidney failure, heart failure, venous insufficiency, and nephrotic syndrome can be confused with angioedema, which is non-pitting. Such conditions often cause edema most prominently in gravity-dependent areas such as the feet and legs, whereas angioedema is not gravity-dependent. Superior vena cava syndrome can cause localized edema of the arm, neck and face. Skin conditions such as contact dermatitis can result in notable edema, as can bacterial skin infections, but are accompanied by skin changes such as papules, plaques, or vesicles.[7]

TREATMENT

The treatment for angioedema with urticaria and for allergic/histaminergic angioedema is as described for urticaria above, although glucocorticoids are often used

Table 3 Differential diagnoses for angioedema	
Condition	Notes
Cellulitis	Erythema, maculopapular or plaques, fever
Dermatitis	Erythema, maculopapular/plaques or vesicles, distribution
Heart failure	Pitting, gravity-dependent, JVD, cardiovascular history, dyspnea, heart sounds, elevated BNP
Hyperthyroidism/proptosis	Periocular changes
Hypoalbuminemia	Pitting, low albumin levels
Kidney failure	Pitting, gravity-dependent, elevated BUN/creatinine
Liver failure	Pitting, gravity-dependent, ascites, stigmata of liver failure, LFT abnormalities
Lipedema	Non-pitting, symmetric excess fat deposition in extremities (especially legs) sparing hands and feet, almost exclusively occurs in women
Lymphedema	Non-pitting, involves extremity (usually one), chronic, postsurgical
Myxedematous hypothyroidism	Non-pitting, TSH/T4 abnormalities, fatigue, cold intolerance, hair loss, constipation, weight gain, thyromegaly may be present
Nephrotic syndrome	Marked proteinuria, insidious onset, fatigue, elevated creatinine
Superior vena cava syndrome	Extremity, neck, and face
Systemic amyloidosis	Macroglossia may be confused with tongue edema
Venous insufficiency	Pitting, gravity-dependent, skin changes, chronic

Abbreviations: BNP, B-type naturetic peptid; JVD, jugular vein distention; LFT, liver function test.
Adapted from Axelrod S, Davis-Lorton M. Urticaria and angioedema. Mt Sinai J Med. 2011;78(5):784-802.

concomitantly with antihistamines at presentation. If airway compromise is threatened due to oral or laryngeal angioedema, intramuscular epinephrine should be used, and intubation may be necessary. Patients on ACE inhibitors presenting with angioedema without urticaria should stop those medications and they should not be restarted. Bradykinin-induced angioedema will not respond to antihistamines. Purified C1 inhibitor concentrate (and other specialty medications) may be used in such cases, in which case specialist referral may be appropriate for such measures.[7,22] In acquired C1 esterase inhibitor deficiency, the underlying cause such as lymphoma or connective tissue disease should be treated and often results in resolution of symptoms.

SUMMARY

Angioedema presents as localized non-pitting edema that may be warm and painful, with or without urticaria. It is typically caused by mast cell release of inflammatory mediators in the lower dermis or subdermis. In such cases it is treated with antihistamines and glucocorticoids. It can also be due to increased bradykinin levels, most commonly due to ACE inhibitors.

CLINICS CARE POINTS

- Acute urticaria can be rapid in onset and last for up to 6 weeks.
- Acute urticaria can be a sign of anaphylaxis.
- Identification and avoidance of triggers is the first line of defense in the treatment of urticaria.
- Second-generation antihistamines at higher than regular dosing is the initial treatment for acute urticaria.
- Chronic urticaria is defined by recurrent crops of urticaria for most days for 6 weeks or longer.
- There are several subtypes of chronic urticaria that should be differentiated.
- Second-generation antihistamines are the initial treatment of choice. Monoclonal antibodies are becoming second-line therapy.
- Angioedema of the tongue or upper airway can be a medical emergency.
- The absence of urticaria or signs of allergic reaction should increase suspicion of bradykinin induced angioedema, often due to angiotensin-converting enzyme inhibitors.
- Treatment in most cases is as with urticaria, with additional attention to airway management if appropriate.

DISCLOSURE

The authors have nothing to disclose.

REFERENCES

1. American Osteopathic College of Dermatology (AOCD). Urticaria. 2011. Available at: https://www.aocd.org/?page=Urticaria%22. Accessed July 7, 2022.
2. Urticaria (hives). NHS inform. 2022. Available at: https://www.nhsinform.scot/illnesses-and-conditions/skin-hair-and-nails/urticaria-hives. Accessed July 7, 2022.
3. Stacey S, Burke D, Brininger T. Urticaria: diagnosis and treatment with osteopathic considerations. Osteopathic Fam Physician 2020;12(3).

4. Schaefer P. Acute and chronic urticaria: evaluation and treatment. Am Fam Physician 2017;95(11):717–24.
5. Schaefer P. Urticaria: evaluation and treatment. Am Fam Physician 2011;83(9): 1078–84.
6. Fonacier L, Dreskin S, Leung D. Primer on allergic and immunologic diseases. J Allergy Clin Immunol 2010;125(2):S138–82.
7. Axelrod S, Davis-Lorton M. Urticaria and angioedema. Mt Sinai J Med 2011;78: 784–802.
8. Abrams EM, Sicherer SH. Diagnosis and management of food allergy. CMAJ 2016;188(15):1087–93.
9. Kayiran MA, Akdeniz N. Diagnosis and treatment of urticaria in primary care. North Clin Istanb 2019;6(1):93–9.
10. Greiwe J, Bernstein JA. Approach to the patient with hives. Med Clin North Am 2020;104(1):15–24.
11. Grattan CEH, Sabroe RA, Greaves MW. Chronic urticaria. J Am Acad Dermatol 2002;46(5):645–60.
12. Sachdeva S, Gupta V, Amin SS, et al. Chronic urticaria. Indian J Dermatol 2011; 56(6):622–8.
13. Leznoff A, Josse RG, Denburg J, et al. Association of chronic urticaria and angioedema with thyroid autoimmunity. Arch Dermatol 1983;119:636–40.
14. Wisnieski JJ. Urticarial vasculitis. Curr Opin Rheumatol 2000;12(1):24–31.
15. Ghiordanescu IM, Ali S, Bumbacea RS. PD31 - Pseudoallergic reactions to food and drugs in children with chronic idiopathic urticaria. Clin Transl Allergy 2014; 4:P31.
16. Buhner S, Reese I, Kuehl F, et al. Pseudoallergic reactions in chronic urticaria are associated with altered gastroduodenal permeability. Allergy 2004;59(10): 1118–23.
17. Beltrani VS. An overview of chronic urticaria. Clin Rev Allergy Immunol 2002; 23(2):147–69.
18. Matos AL, Figueiredo C, Gonçalo M. Differential diagnosis of urticarial lesions. Front Allergy 2022;3. https://doi.org/10.3389/falgy.2022.808543.
19. Kolkhir P, Altrichter S, Munoz M, et al. New treatments for chronic urticaria. Ann Allergy Asthma Immunol 2020;124(1):2–12.
20. Bernstein JA, Lang DM, Khan DA, et al. The diagnosis and management of acute and chronic urticaria: 2014 update. J Allergy Clin Immunol 2014;133(5):1270–7.
21. Zuberbier T, Abdul Latiff AH, Abuzakouk M, et al. The international EAACI/GA[2]-LEN/EuroGuiDerm/APAAACI guideline for the definition, classification, diagnosis, and management of urticaria. Allergy 2022;77(3):734–66.
22. Macy E. Practical management of new-onset urticaria and angioedema presenting in primary care, urgent care, and the emergency department. Perm J 2021; 25:21–058.

Inborn Errors of Immunity

Carolyn H. Baloh[a],*, Hey Chong[b]

KEYWORDS

- Immunodeficiency • Antibody deficiency • Combined immunodeficiency
- Inborn errors of immunity • Recurrent infection(s) • Immunoglobulin replacement
- Antibiotic prophylaxis • Hematopoietic stem cell transplantation

KEY POINTS

- Inborn errors of immunity (IEIs) are caused by genetic mutations that result in an increased frequency and/or severity of infections, immune dysregulation, autoimmunity, and/or malignancy.
- A delay in detecting IEIs has been shown to have adverse consequences for patients; therefore, a PCP should be familiar with key features of IEIs and have a low threshold for referral.
- Laboratory evaluation for IEIs assess whether certain parts of the immune system are present and whether they are functioning properly.
- Treatment of IEIs can include prophylactic antibiotics, hematopoietic stem cell transplantation, gene therapy, and targeted biologics, depending on the specific diagnosis.

INTRODUCTION

Inborn errors of immunity (IEIs) are a category of medical diagnoses caused by genetic mutations that result in an increased frequency and/or severity of infections, immune dysregulation, autoimmunity, and/or malignancy.[1] IEIs are estimated to occur in 1 in 1000 to 1 in 5000 individuals.[1,2] They can present at any age, with specific diagnoses being more predominant in certain age groups. Presenting features can be an abnormal newborn screen, increased frequency and/or severity of infections, autoimmunity, immune dysregulation, and/or malignancy. Detection of these IEIs requires a thorough medical history screening for infections and evidence of immune dysfunction (eg, recurrent fevers, autoimmunity) as well as a physical examination screening for

[a] Division of Allergy and Clinical Immunology, Department of Medicine, Harvard Medical School, Brigham and Women's Hospital, 60 Fenwood Road, BTM/Hale Building, 5th Floor, Boston, MA 02115, USA; [b] Division of Allergy and Immunology, Department of Pediatrics, UPMC Children's Hospital of Pittsburgh, 4401 Penn Avenue, AOB 3300, Pittsburgh, PA 15224, USA
* Corresponding author. Division of Allergy and Clinical Immunology, Department of Medicine, Harvard Medical School, Brigham and Women's Hospital, 60 Fenwood Road, BTM/Hale Building, 5th Floor, Boston, MA 02115, USA
E-mail address: cbaloh@bwh.harvard.edu

Prim Care Clin Office Pract 50 (2023) 253–268
https://doi.org/10.1016/j.pop.2022.12.001
0095-4543/23/© 2022 Elsevier Inc. All rights reserved.
primarycare.theclinics.com

current infection(s), sequelae of infections, and evidence of immune dysfunction (eg, enlarged lymph nodes, enteropathy, endocrinopathies). Laboratory evaluation of the immune system is based on the suspected diagnosis and can include evaluation of antibody number and function, immune cell frequency and function, and the complement pathway. Treatment varies from prophylactic antibiotics to hematopoietic stem cells transplantation. In this article, we will present an overview of IEIs with a focus on key points for the primary care provider (PCP).

DEFINITIONS

IEIs can be subdivided into primary immunodeficiency diseases (PIDDs) and primary immune regulatory disorders (PIRDs). PIDDs are a category of diagnoses where the predominant feature is recurrent and/or severe infections. Patients with PIDDs also have a predisposition to immune dysregulation, autoimmunity, and malignancy. PIDDs can be further subdivided into categories including combined immunodeficiency (CID), predominantly antibody deficiencies (PADs), primary phagocytic disorders, complement deficiencies, and others[3] (Table 1). CIDs are diseases of lymphocyte number and/or function, which affect predominantly T cells and can also affect B and/or NK cells. They are typically the most severe PIDDs and can present with viral, fungal, and bacterial infections. PADs are diseases in which B cell and/or antibody number or function are abnormal resulting in recurrent sinopulmonary infections. Primary phagocytic disorders are characterized by abnormal phagocyte (neutrophil, macrophage, or dendritic cell) number and/or function leading to recurrent skin infections and abscesses of internal organs. Complement deficiencies have either absent or abnormally functioning component(s) of the complement system. These can present with an increased risk of Neisserial or pyogenic infections, a lupus-like syndrome, or atypical hemolytic uremic syndrome (aHUS).[3]

In recent years, PIRDs have arisen as a new category of diagnoses where the primary feature is immune dysfunction, and a secondary feature is immunodeficiency. Immune dysfunction can include autoinflammation/hyperinflammation, autoimmunity, lymphoproliferation, malignancy, and severe atopy[4] (Table 2).

The International Union of Immunological Societies Expert Committee (IUIS) has generated a document detailing all known genetic causes of IEIs (PIDDs and PIRDs).[3] More than 400 genetic causes of IEIs have been identified, with more causes being frequently identified.[3,5] There are still some IEIs for which we have not identified the causative genetic mutation (eg, common variable immunodeficiency [CVID]). A subset of IEIs is detailed in Tables 1 and 2. These tables are not meant to be a comprehensive listing but rather to familiarize the PCP with some of the most common diagnoses, most serious diagnoses, and to gain a sense of the breadth of different diseases in this area. Additional IEIs can be found in the IUIS document.[3]

DIAGNOSIS
History

A delay in diagnosis of an IEI has been shown to correlate with poorer outcomes.[6] Therefore, it is essential for the PCP to be aware of elements of the medical history concerning for IEI. In 1993, a group of experts convened and developed "10 warning signs" of PIDD (Table 3). These have been published by the Jeffrey Model Foundation and are widely used to help PCP's know when to refer patients for evaluation.[7,8] Evaluation is recommended if 2 or more signs are positive. Although these have been helpful in promoting awareness of PIDDs, several studies have called into question their lack of validation.[9-11] The sensitivity of these criteria has been estimated to be 63%

Table 1
Key features of a subset of primary immunodeficiency diseases

Diagnosis	Genetics	Key Features
CIDs		
SCID	IL2RG, JAK3, IL7R, CD3D, CD3E, CD3Z, PTPRC, LAT, CORO1A, FOXN1, ADA, AK2, RAC2, LIG4, NHEJ1, PRKDC, RAG1, RAG2, DCLRE1C	T cell lymphopenia, often detected by abnormal newborn screen or positive family history, severe infections, oral thrush, intractable diarrhea, pneumonia, failure to thrive, some have syndromic features, requires transplantation or gene therapy to survive beyond first year of life[43]
DGS	22q11.2 deletion, TBX1, 10p13-p14 deletion, CHD7, SEMA3E, 11q23 deletion, FOXN1	Hypoparathyroidism, viral and bacterial infections, congenital heart disease, other syndromic features, approximately 1% have a significant CID and require thymus transplantation while the other 99% have normal to mildly impaired immune systems[44–46]
WAS	WAS	Recurrent viral, fungal, or opportunistic infections, bloody diarrhea, eczema, autoimmunity, malignancy, low antibody levels, inadequate vaccine titers, T cell lymphopenia, anemia, thrombocytopenia[47–49]
A-T	ATM	Ataxia, telangiectasias, pulmonary infections, malignancy, radiosensitivity[50]
HIES	STAT3, ZNF34, SPINK5, PGM3, CARD11, ERBB21P, IL6R, IL6ST, TGFBR1, TGFBR2	Increased incidence of atopy, skin infections, respiratory infections, abscesses without pus, musculoskeletal abnormalities, elevated IgE levels[2,51]
PADs		
CVID	PIK3CD, PIK3Ra, PTEN, ARHGEF, SH3KBP1, SEC61A1, RAC2, CD20, TNFRSF13 B, TNFRSF13 C, TNFSF12, IRF2BP2, CD19, CD81, CD21, TRNT1, NFKB1, NFKB2, IKZF1, ATP6AP1, GCS1	Recurrent sinopulmonary infections, autoimmunity, malignancy, low IgG with low IgA and/or IgM, inadequate vaccine titers[52]
XLA	BTK	Recurrent infections with encapsulated bacteria early in life, diarrhea, enteroviral meningitis, autoimmunity, malignancy, absence of B cells and antibodies[53]

(continued on next page)

Table 1
(continued)

Diagnosis	Genetics	Key Features
IGAD	Unknown genetic cause	Low or absent IgA, normal IgG and IgM, 85%–90% are asymptomatic, 10%–15% have sinopulmonary infections, gastrointestinal infections, autoimmunity, atopy[54,55]
Hyper IgM syndrome	AICDA, UNG, INO80, MSH6	Sinopulmonary infections, opportunistic infections, enlarged lymph nodes, malignancy, normal or elevated IgM, low IgG, A, E[49,56]
SAD	Unknown genetic cause	Recurrent respiratory infections, normal antibody levels, inadequate polysaccharide pneumococcal vaccine titers[20,57]
THI	Unknown genetic cause	Can be asymptomatic or have recurrent sinopulmonary infections, self-resolves by 2–5 y of age[58]
Predominantly Phagocytic Disorders		
CGD	CYBB, NCF1, CYBA, NCF4, NCF2, CYBC1	Visceral abscesses, fungal infections, cellulitis, lymphadenitis, failure to thrive, granulomas[59,60]
LAD	ITGB2, SLC35C1, FERMT3	Omphalitis, periodontitis, recurrent infections, dysmorphic features, bleeding disorders[61]
GATA2 deficiency	GATA2	Recurrent infections, lymphedema, lymphoma, cytopenias, and alveolar proteinosis[62]
Complement Deficiencies		
High susceptibility to infections	C3, C5, C6, C7, C8A, C8B, C8G, C9, PFC, CFD, MASP2, FCN3, CFB	Can be associated with disseminated Neisserial infections or recurrent pyogenic infections[2,63]
Low susceptibility to infections	C1QA, C1QB, C1QC, C1R, C1S, C2, C4A + C4B, C3, CFB, CFH, CFHR1-5, THBD, CD46, SERPING1, CD59, CD55	Can be associated with an SLE-like syndrome and infections with encapsulated organisms (C1, C2, C4, or MBL deficiency) or with aHUS (Factor H or CD46 deficiency)[2,63]

Abbreviations: A-T, Ataxia-telangectasia; CGD, Chronic granulomatous disease; CVID, Common variable immunodeficiency; DGS, DiGeorge Syndrome; HIeS, Hyper-IgE syndromes; IGAD, IgA deficiency; LAD, Leukocyte adhesion deficiency; MBL, Mannose binding lectin; SAD, Specific antibody deficiency; SCID, Severe combined immunodeficiency; THI, Transient hypogammaglobulinemia of infancy; WAS, Wiskott-Aldrich Syndrome; XLA, X-linked agammaglobulinemia.

Table 2
Key features of a subset of primary immune regulatory disorders

Diagnosis	Genetics	Key Features
Syndromes with Autoimmunity		
Autoimmune lymphoproliferative syndrome (ALPS)	TNFRSF6, TNFSF6, CASP10, CASP8, FADD	Chronic lymphadenopathy and/or splenomegaly, cytopenias, lymphoma[64]
APECED	AIRE	Chronic mucocutaneous candidiasis, polyendocrinopathy, dystrophy of nails and dental enamel lung disease[65]
IPEX	FOXP3	Presents very early in life, autoimmune enteropathy (presenting with watery diarrhea), autoimmune endocrinopathy (type 1 diabetes), dermatitis, atopy, recurrent infections[33,66]
Diseases with susceptibility to HLH		
Chediak Higashi syndrome	LYST	Partial oculocutaneous albinism, silvery hair, bleeding diathesis, neurologic deficits, recurrent pyogenic infections[41]
Griscelli syndrome, type 2	RAB27 A	Silvery hair, neurologic deficits, fever, hepatosplenomegaly, cytopenias[3,39]
Hermansky-Pudlak syndrome, types 2 or 10	AP3B1	Oculocutaneous albinism, bleeding diathesis, pulmonary fibrosis, nystagmus, seizures, developmental delay, hearing loss, neutropenia[3,40]
Familial HLH syndromes	PRF1, UNC13D, STX11, STXBP2, FAAP24, SLC7A7	Inherited predisposition to develop HLH, fever, hepatosplenomegaly, cytopenias[3]
Autoinflammatory syndromes		
Familial Mediterranean Fever (FMF)	MEFV	Episodes of inflammation (fever, polyserositis, rash) lasting 1–4 d occurring with variable frequency, amyloidosis[3,31]
TNF receptor-associated periodic syndrome (TRAPS)	TNFRSF1A	Episodes of inflammation (fever, migratory inflammation, conjunctivitis) lasting 1–4 wk occurring with variable frequency, amyloidosis[3,31]
Familial cold autoinflammatory syndrome (CAPS)	NLRP3, NRLP12	Episodes of inflammation (nonpruritic urticaria, arthritis, fever) triggered by cold and lasting 1–2 d [3,67]

Abbreviations: APECED, Autoimmune polyendocrinopathy-candidiasis-ectodermal dystrophy; IPEX, Immunodysregulation polyendocrinopathy enteropathy X-linked; HLH, Hemophagocytic lymphohistiocytosis; TNF, Tumor necrosis factor.

to 64%.[9,11] The specific criteria of having a positive family history of PIDD, history of receiving intravenous (IV) antibiotics for sepsis, and failure to thrive have been present in at least 89% of patients with CIDs, phagocytic disorders, and complement deficiency.[10] None of the criteria has detected a large percentage of patients with PADs.[10] Additionally, it has been suggested that different criteria altogether are

Table 3
Jeffrey Model Foundation 10 warning signs of primary immunodeficiency

Children (up to 18 Year Old)	Adults
≥4 ear infections within 1 y	≥2 ear infections within 1 y
≥2 serious sinus infections within 1 y	≥2 serious sinus infections within 1 y, in the absence of allergy
≥2 pneumonias in 1 y	1 pneumonia per year for >1 y
≥2 mo on antibiotics with little effect	Chronic diarrhea with weight loss
Need for IV antibiotics to clear infections	Recurrent need for IV antibiotics to clear infections
Recurrent, deep skin or organ abscesses	Recurrent, deep skin or organ abscesses
Persistent thrush in mouth or fungal infection on skin	Persistent thrush in mouth or fungal infection on skin or elsewhere
A family history of primary immunodeficiency	A family history of primary immunodeficiency
≥2 deep-seated infections including septicemia	Infection with a normal harmless tuberculosis-like bacteria
Failure of an infant to gain weight or grow normally	Recurrent viral infections (colds, herpes, warts, condyloma)

needed for children compared with adults. The most relevant criteria for children have been suggested to be recurrent pneumonia, failure to thrive, need for IV antibiotics, serious bacterial infection, and recurrent otitis media. Although for adults, recurrent otitis media, recurrent sinusitis, diarrhea with weight loss, and recurrent viral infection were the most useful criteria.[9] This is likely reflective of the fact that CIDs are more common in children and PADs become more common in adult patients.

Additionally, PIRDs were not a known disease category when the warning signs were created. Patients with PIRDs, and some PIDDs, can present with autoinflammation/hyperinflammation, autoimmunity, lymphoproliferation, malignancy, and/or severe atopy before they develop recurrent and/or severe infections.[4] PCPs should familiarize themselves with key features of IEIs and have a low threshold for referring patients for evaluation, recognizing that no criteria are perfect.

In addition to components of the history guiding who should be referred for IEI evaluation, there are components that are useful for identifying the specific diagnosis. Age can be an important clue to diagnosis with the most severe immunodeficiencies presenting as early as the first weeks of life.[12] Antibody deficiencies typically do not present until at least 6 months of age when the maternal antibodies wane and can present through adulthood.[12,13] Family history of IEI, malignancy, autoimmunity, lymphoproliferation, and unexplained deaths are also key red flags for IEI and should be recorded.[10] It is important to gather as much information about previous and current infections as possible including the site of infection, pathogen(s), treatment(s), duration, and severity (**Table 4**).[1,13] Additionally, identification of comorbid diagnoses (especially autoimmunity, malignancy, and atopy) and previous reactions to vaccines or transfusions are useful in identifying a specific diagnosis.[12,13]

Physical Examination

A thorough physical examination is a part of the evaluation for IEIs. An examination should include an assessment of constitutional features including weight gain/loss and height, manifestations of current/previous infections, and other organ-specific

Table 4
Common infections associated with inborn errors of immunity

IEI Category	Pathogens
CIDs	Encapsulated bacteria (*Streptococcus pneumoniae, Haemophilus influenzae*) Fungus (*Candida* species) Viruses (CMV, EBV, RSV, VZV, HSV, measles, influenza, parainfluenza) Mycobacteria Opportunistic organisms (*P jirovecii* (PJP), *Cryptosporidium* species) Attenuated vaccines may cause infection (oral polio, rotavirus, varicella, BCG)
PADs	Encapsulated bacteria (*S pneumoniae, H influenzae*) Parasites (*Giardia lamblia*) *Enterovirus* species Atypical bacteria (*Mycoplasma* species, *Ureaplasma* species) Causes of infectious diarrhea include *G lamblia, Salmonella enterica, Campylobacter jejuni, Norovirus, Cryptosporidium* species, *Mycoplasma* species, and *Enterovirus* species Certain types of HIGM can have opportunistic and viral infections
Primary Phagocytic Disorders	Gram negative bacteria (*Escherichia coli, Burkholderia cepacia* complex, *Serratia marcescens*) *Staphylococcus aureus* Fungal infections (*Aspergillus* species, *Nocardia* species) GATA2 can also present with HPV
Complement Deficiencies	Encapsulated bacteria (*S pneumoniae, H influenzae*) *Neisseria* species
PIRDs	APECED—*Candida albicans* IPEX—*Enterococcus faecalis, Staphylococcus* species, CMV, *C albicans* Chediak Higashi Syndrome—pyogenic infections

Abbreviations: CMV, cytomegalovirus; BCG, bacille Calmette-Guerin; EBV, epstein-barr virus; HPV, human papillomavirus; HSV, herpes simplex virus; RSV, respiratory syncytial virus; VZV, varicella zoster virus.

features (**Table 5**).[12] It is also essential to examine for the absence of lymphoid tissue (ie, tonsils, lymph nodes) because this can be a clue that the patient does not have B cells.[12]

Laboratory Evaluation for Combined Immunodeficiencies

As of 2019, the newborn screen in all 50 states includes the T cell receptor excision circle severe combined immunodeficiency (SCID) screen.[14] This screen detects T cell lymphopenia. It is *critical* for patients with a positive screen to be referred to an immunologist as soon as possible for immunologic and diagnostic workup.[15] An abnormal SCID screen result could indicate one of several PIDs or PIRDs with T cell lymphopenia including DiGeorge syndrome (DGS), Trisomy 21, ataxia telangectasia (A-T), secondary T cell lymphopenia, and prematurity.[14] Primary care physicians are often the first to notify patients of these abnormal SCID screen results. Patients should not be told that they have SCID but rather lymphopenia, and that further workup is needed.

A complete blood count with differential can be used to screen for lymphopenia in patients of all ages. Additional laboratory evaluation for CIDs includes flow cytometry

Table 5
Key physical examination features and corresponding inborn errors of immunity

Feature	IEI
General	CIDs
Failure to thrive	FMF, TRAPS, CAPS
Fever	
Head, eyes, ears, nose, throat	DGS, LAD
Dysmorphic facial features	SCID, HIES, APECED
Oral thrush	A-T
Eye telangiectasias	Hermansky-Pudlak syndrome
Nystagmus	PADs
Tympanic membrane scarring	Chediak Higashi syndrome, Hermansky-Pudlak syndrome
Oculocutaneous albinism	Chediak Higashi syndrome, Griscelli syndrome
Silvery hair	
Lymphoid tissues	XLA
Absent lymphoid tissue	HIGM, ALPS, CVID, ALPS, Familial HLH syndromes
Lymph node hyperplasia	
Cardiac	DGS
Congenital heart disease	
Pulmonary	PADs
Rales/rhonchi/digital clubbing	
Abdominal	PADs, ALPS, Familial HLH syndromes
Hepatomegaly/splenomegaly	LAD
Omphalitis	WAS
Bloody diarrhea	SCID, IPEX
Watery diarrhea	
Skin	WAS, IPEX
Dermatitis/eczema	FMF
Sunburn-like rash	APECED
Dystrophy of nails/teeth	HIES
Cold abscesses	CAPS
Urticaria	
Musculoskeletal	Complement deficiencies
Lupus-like features	HIES
Fractures	HIES
Scoliosis	

to enumerate T, B, and NK cells; proliferation to mitogens and antigens (a measure of T cell function); NK cell function test; and genetic testing. Genetic testing is pursued if it will help to ensure a correct diagnosis and if it can expand treatment options to include targeted therapies and/or hematopoietic stem cell transplantation (HSCT). Evaluation of B cells and antibodies (see later discussion) should also be performed when there is concern for a CID.

Laboratory Evaluation for Predominantly Antibody Deficiencies

As part of the evaluation for PADs, it is useful to examine the presence or absence of antibodies as well as their function. Levels of IgG, IgA, IgM, and IgE can be measured with nephelometry and function can be assessed using vaccine titers. Normal levels of IgG, IgA, IgM, and IgE vary by age, so appropriate reference values must be used. Abnormal results can indicate the presence of a PAD, CID, or can be the result of another medical problem. Secondary causes of low antibody levels include burns/trauma, gastrointestinal loss, nephrotic syndrome, malignancy, and certain medications.[16]

Vaccine-specific antibody titers can be assessed in patients aged 2 years and older who have completed their primary vaccination series as recommended by the Centers for Disease Control (CDC). Titers should be checked to vaccines that require T cell help (tetanus, diphtheria, and pneumococcal conjugate vaccine [PCV13]) and to those that are T cell independent (pneumovax [PPV23]).[1,17] Interpretation of tetanus and diphtheria titers should be done using the normal ranges provided by the laboratory. Pneumococcal titers should be checked to 23 serotypes. A pneumovax (PPV23) is often administered as part of the evaluative process in patients over a year of age.[1,17] Interpretation of pneumococcal titers is age dependent with an adequate response generally defined as

- In a child aged younger than 6 years: 50% or greater of the serotypes have titers that are 1.3 μg/mL or greater.
- In a child aged older than 6 years or an adult: 75% or greater of the serotypes have titers that are 1.3 μg/mL or greater.[17]

It is normal for antibody responses to vaccines to wane over time, and a booster vaccine may be needed to confirm whether antibody function is adequate. If a pneumovax or a booster of tetanus or diphtheria is administered, the optimal time to check titers is 4 to 6 weeks after administration.[1,17]

Additional testing that may be sent during the evaluation for PADs include flow cytometry for T, B, and NK cells; flow cytometry for B cell subsets; and genetic testing.

Laboratory Evaluation for Phagocytic (Neutrophilic Defects)

A CBC with differential including manual review of the blood smear is a useful first step in ensuring that neutrophils are present in adequate number and morphology. Additional laboratory evaluation includes an oxidative burst test, a measure of neutrophil function, and genetic testing.

Laboratory Evaluation for Complement Disorders

First-line tests for the evaluation of a complement disorder include a complement activity, Total (CH50) and an complement activity, Total (CH50). These provide information regarding whether the classical or alternative pathways, respectively, are functioning appropriately. Additional evaluation can include the measurement of specific complement protein levels and genetic testing.

THERAPEUTIC OPTIONS
Antibiotic Prophylaxis

Antibiotic prophylaxis can be useful for many different IEIs.[1,18] Choice of antibiotic agent should be based on diagnosis, infection history, guidelines and in the absence of guidelines expert experience/consensus.[1,18] Common regimens are listed in **Table 6**. There is currently debate among experts regarding the utility of antibiotic prophylaxis versus immunoglobulin replacement for PADs and no controlled studies exist.[1,18,19] Mild PADs including symptomatic transient hypogammaglobulinemia of infancy (THI) and symptomatic IgA deficiency (IGAD) can generally be managed with prophylactic antibiotics.[18] Antibiotic prophylaxis and immunoglobulin replacement are both used in X-linked agammaglobulinemia (XLA) and specific antibody deficiency (SAD) depending on disease severity and immunologist preference.[18,20–22] CVID is typically managed with immunoglobulin replacement but antibiotics can be useful for breakthrough infections despite adequate immunoglobulin replacement.[1]

Table 6
Commonly used antibiotic regimens for patients with primarily antibody deficiencies to prevent sinopulmonary infections

Antibiotic (Oral)	Regimen for Children	Regimen for Adults
Oral agents		
Amoxicillin (consider with clavulanate if necessary)	10–20 mg/kg daily or twice daily	500–1000 mg daily or twice daily
Trimethoprime (TMP)/ sulfamethoxazole (dosing for TMP)	5 mg/kg daily or twice daily	160 mg daily or twice daily
Azithromycin	10 mg/kg weekly or 5 mg/kg every other day	500 mg weekly or 250 mg every other day
Clarithromycin	7.5 mg/kg daily or twice daily	500 mg daily or twice daily
Doxycycline	Age >8 y: 25–50 mg daily or twice daily	100 mg daily or twice daily
Inhaled agents		
Gentamycin	Age >6y: 80 mg twice daily, 28 days on, 28 days off OR: 21 days on 7 days off	
Tobramycin	Age >6y: 300 mg twice daily, 28 days on, 28 days off	

Additional options are available if these regimens fail to work or if a patient becomes resistant.
From Bonilla FA, Khan DA, Ballas ZK, et al. Practice parameter for the diagnosis and management of primary immunodeficiency. J Allergy Clin Immunol. 2015;136(5):1186-205.e2078.

An important consideration when using prophylactic antibiotics is the potential to induce antibiotic resistance. Therefore, when prophylaxis is used, it is common to rotate antibiotics but there is no clear data supporting this practice.[19] Fortunately, there have been no published cases of infections from resistant organisms in patients receiving antibiotic prophylaxis for PADs.[1] Other potential concerns include induction of antibiotic hypersensitivity, *Clostridium difficile* infection, and alteration of the gut microbiome.[19]

Prophylaxis is important to prevent life-threating infections with *Pneumocystis jirovecii* (PJP), virus, and fungi in patients with CIDs. PJP prophylaxis is required for SCID, DGS (only when T cells are significantly low), Wiskott-Aldrich syndrome (WAS), A-T, and hyper-IgE syndromes (HIES).[18] Patients with SCID and HIES also require prophylaxis against fungal infections.[18] Patients with SCID should receive prophylaxis to prevent herpes virus infections.[18] Patients with PIDs and PIRDs who have had a splenectomy should receive penicillin to prevent infections with encapsulated organisms.[18] Antibiotic prophylaxis in patients with CIDs is often used as a bridge to prevent serious infection before a more definitive therapy such as HSCT.

Prophylactic antibiotics have a role in many other PIDDs. Antibiotic prophylaxis can prevent recurrent bacterial infections in chronic granulomatous disease (CGD) and leukocyte adhesion deficiency (LAD), fungal infections in CGD, and Neisserial infections in complement deficiencies.[18] Antibiotic prophylaxis in these patients can be either life-long or as a bridge to a more definitive therapy.

Immunoglobulin Replacement

Immunoglobulin replacement is a cornerstone of therapy for PADs. Immunoglobulin replacement has been shown to prevent infections including pneumonia, serious bacterial illness, and enteroviral meningoencephalitis in patients with PADs.[23–25] There are many products available for immunoglobulin replacement, and the choice of the product should be a shared process with the patient and based on lifestyle preferences, side effects, and comorbidities.[23,26] Both subcutaneous immunoglobulin (SCIG) and intravenous immunoglobulin (IVIG) can be used in babies, children, and adults. Immunoglobulin replacement can safely be given to patients deficient in IgA.[23]

IV products are typically administered every 3 to 4 weeks in an infusion center and have been used regularly since the 1980s. They have been associated with larger variance in IgG levels in the blood stream and this can lead to adverse effects. Common side effects, occurring in 5% to 15% of infusions, include headache, fever, chills, flushing, rash, breathing difficulties, abdominal pain, arthralgias, myalgias, anxiety, and malaise.[23,27] Most adverse reactions occur during either the first IVIG infusion, when a change in product is made, or when there is underlying chronic inflammation.[23] Less common, occurring in 1% of patients are the more severe possible side effects including renal failure, thrombosis (black box warning), and aseptic meningitis. Therefore, care in product choice and dosing is particularly important in patients with kidney disease, diabetes, and/or a history of thrombotic events.[23,26,27] Another more recently recognized side effect has been wear-off effect. The wear-off effect occurs when the circulating IgG level falls in the approximately 1 week before the next infusion. It is characterized by fatigue, malaise, arthralgias, myalgias, and increased rates of infection.[28,29]

Subcutaneous products were first approved in the United States in 2006 and can be administered at home on a weekly basis. They have a lower incidence of side effects and wear-off syndromes due to the steadier IgG concentration in the blood stream.[23] The most common adverse reaction to SCIG is a localized site reaction.[23]

Dosing should be adjusted based on efficacy in an individual patient. Maintaining a trough level greater than 800 mg/dL has been shown to prevent serious bacterial illness and enteroviral meningoencephalitis.[30] Multiple studies, including a meta-analysis, support that a goal trough of 1000 mg/dL is optimal to prevent pneumonia.[24,25]

Immunoglobulin replacement can also be useful in other IEIs as a lifelong infection prevention measure or as a bridge to a more definitive therapy.

Immunomodulation

PIRDs are often managed by using an immunomodulatory agent(s). Historically, immunomodulatory agents have had broad impacts on the immune system. More recently, targeted agents have been developed. Our field is working to move to an approach where we are modulating the specific pathway affected by the genetic mutation. For example, patients with autoinflammatory syndromes often have excessive production of interleukin-1 (IL-1) by the inflammasome and can benefit from IL-1 antagonists.[31] Janus kinase (JAK) inhibitors are currently under investigation for autoimmune polyendocrinopathy candidiasis ectodermal dystrophy (APECED).[32] Many different immunomodulators have been used to treat Immunodysregulation polyendocrinopathy enteropathy X-linked (IPEX) and APECED without consensus for an optimal approach.[33,34]

Hematopoietic Stem Cell Transplantation

HSCT is a definitive therapy for many CIDs, phagocytic defects, and PIRDs. In general, the younger a patient is when they undergo HSCT, the better the outcome. This is particularly important for patients with SCID who require bone marrow transplant or gene therapy to survive past 1 year of age. While they are awaiting HSCT, they should

1. *Not* receive live vaccines, including rotavirus
2. Receive PJP and fungal prophylaxis
3. Receive immunoglobulin replacement

4. Discontinue breast feeding until it is known if mother is cytomegalovirus (CMV) positive
5. If blood transfusion is required, products should be irradiated, CMV negative, and leukoreduced.[35]

Overall survival of a patient with SCID who has received a bone marrow transplant in the United States between 2010 and 2014 is approximately 90% at 2 years of age.[36] The most significant predictors of poor outcome are pretransplant infection and increased age at transplant.[37,38]

Bone marrow transplantation may also be available on a clinical or research basis for other PIDDs (eg, WAS, CGD, LAD, HIES, HIGM) and PIRDs (eg, IPEX and diseases with increased risk of hemophagocytic lymphohistiocytosis [HLH]).[1,4,39–41] The decision of whether to proceed with a transplant in non-SCID IEIs usually includes the genetic diagnosis, possible donor(s), age of patient, current/previous infections, likelihood of malignancy, and comorbidities. When conditioning is used, the goal is to balance toxicity with maximizing engraftment.[4] In general, to proceed with transplantation, the risk of the disease, including risk of future malignancy, must outweigh the risk of the transplant.

Gene Therapy

Technology allowing for safe and effective gene therapy for PIDDs has greatly advanced during the last 30 years. The field has developed new viral vectors to prevent leukoproliferative complications and new regimens using reduced intensity conditioning to improve engraftment and limit toxicity.[42] Gene therapy is available on a clinical or research basis for some subtypes of SCID, WAS, LAD, and CGD.[1] Editing of the endogenous gene is also under investigation for some subtypes of SCID, HIGM, CGD, IPEX, and others.[42]

SUMMARY

IEIs encompass a broad range of diagnoses with common features of infection susceptibility and immune dysregulation. PCPs are at the front line for the detection of IEIs and should be familiar with key features and have a low threshold to refer for evaluation. They can also play a role in managing IEIs, especially more mild diagnoses.

CLINICS CARE POINTS

- IEIs are a category of genetic diseases where patients experience recurrent infections, autoinflammation/hyperinflammation, autoimmunity, lymphoproliferation, malignancy, and/or severe atopy. They can be subdivided into PIDDs and PIRDs.
- PCPs should be familiar with key features of IEIs, and if concern for IEI arises based on history, physical examination, and/or bloodwork, a referral to an immunologist should be made.
- A PCP can assist the immunologist in evaluation by obtaining some basic laboratories before referral including a CBC with differential, antibody levels, titers to tetanus, pertussis, and pneumococcus, and possibly additional tests.
- A baby with a family history of SCID, a low absolute lymphocyte count (ALC), and/or an abnormal newborn screen should be referred to an immunologist immediately for diagnosis confirmation and evaluation for HSCT.
- If a PCP is managing a patient with prophylactic antibiotics specific dosing and a rotation between different antibiotics is recommended to achieve maximum efficacy and prevent antibiotic resistance.

DISCLOSURE

The authors have nothing to disclose.

REFERENCES

1. Bonilla FA, Khan DA, Ballas ZK, et al. Practice parameter for the diagnosis and management of primary immunodeficiency. J Allergy Clin Immunol 2015;136(5):1186–205, e1-78.
2. Tangye SG, Al-Herz W, Bousfiha A, et al. Human Inborn Errors of Immunity: 2019 Update on the Classification from the International Union of Immunological Societies Expert Committee. J Clin Immunol 2020;40(1):65.
3. Bousfiha A, Jeddane L, Picard C, et al. Human Inborn Errors of Immunity: 2019 Update of the IUIS Phenotypical Classification. J Clin Immunol 2020;40(1):66–81.
4. Chan AYT TR. Primary immune regulatory disorders: a growing universe of immune dysregulation. Curr Opin Allergy Clin Immunol 2020;20(6):582–90.
5. Tangye SG, Al-Herz W, Bousfiha A, et al. The Ever-Increasing Array of Novel Inborn Errors of Immunity: an Interim Update by the IUIS Committee. J Clin Immunol 2021;41(3):666–79.
6. Waltenburg R, Kobrynski L, Reyes M, et al. Primary immunodeficiency diseases: practice among primary care providers and awareness among the general public, United States, 2008. Genet Med 2010;12(12):792–800.
7. Modell V, Gee B, Lewis DB, et al. Global study of primary immunodeficiency diseases (PI)–diagnosis, treatment, and economic impact: an updated report from the Jeffrey Modell Foundation. Immunol Res 2011;51(1):61–70.
8. Warning Signs of Primary Immunodeficiency. 2022. Available at: http://www.info4pi.org/library/educational-materials/10-warning-signs. Accessed 07 13, 2022.
9. Bjelac JA, Yonkof JR, Fernandez J. Differing Performance of the Warning Signs for Immunodeficiency in the Diagnosis of Pediatric Versus Adult Patients in a Two-Center Tertiary Referral Population. J Clin Immunol 2019;39(1):90–8.
10. Subbarayan A, Colarusso G, Hughes SM, et al. Clinical features that identify children with primary immunodeficiency diseases. Pediatrics 2011;127(5):810–6.
11. MacGinnitie A, Aloi F, Mishra S. Clinical characteristics of pediatric patients evaluated for primary immunodeficiency. Pediatr Allergy Immunol 2011;22(7):671–5.
12. Ballow M. Approach to the patient with recurrent infections. Clin Rev Allergy Immunol 2008;34(2):129–40.
13. Slatter MA, Gennery AR. Clinical immunology review series: an approach to the patient with recurrent infections in childhood. Clin Exp Immunol 2008;152(3):389–96.
14. Currier R, Puck JM. SCID newborn screening: What we've learned. J Allergy Clin Immunol 2021;147(2):417–26.
15. Buckley RH. SCID: A Pediatric Emergency. N C Med J 2019;80(1):55–6.
16. Agarwal S, Cunningham-Rundles C. Assessment and clinical interpretation of reduced IgG values. Ann Allergy Asthma Immunol 2007;99(3):281–3.
17. Orange JS, Ballow M, Stiehm ER, et al. Use and interpretation of diagnostic vaccination in primary immunodeficiency: a working group report of the Basic and Clinical Immunology Interest Section of the American Academy of Allergy, Asthma & Immunology. J Allergy Clin Immunol 2012;130(3 Suppl):S1–24.
18. Kuruvilla M, de la Morena MT. Antibiotic prophylaxis in primary immune deficiency disorders. J Allergy Clin Immunol Pract 2013;1(6):573–82.

19. Ballow M, Paris K, de la Morena M. Should Antibiotic Prophylaxis Be Routinely Used in Patients with Antibody-Mediated Primary Immunodeficiency? J Allergy Clin Immunol Pract 2018;6(2):421–6.

20. Joud H, Nguyen AL, Constantine G, et al. Prophylactic Antibiotics Versus Immunoglobulin Replacement in Specific Antibody Deficiency. J Clin Immunol 2020; 40(1):158–64.

21. Smits BM, Kleine Budde I, de Vries E, et al. Immunoglobulin Replacement Therapy Versus Antibiotic Prophylaxis as Treatment for Incomplete Primary Antibody Deficiency. J Clin Immunol 2021;41(2):382–92.

22. Pandya A, Burgen E, Chen GJ, et al. Comparison of management options for specific antibody deficiency. Allergy Asthma Proc 2021;42(1):87–92.

23. Perez EE, Orange JS, Bonilla F, et al. Update on the use of immunoglobulin in human disease: A review of evidence. J Allergy Clin Immunol 2017;139(3S):S1–46.

24. Orange JS, Grossman WJ, Navickis RJ, et al. Impact of trough IgG on pneumonia incidence in primary immunodeficiency: A meta-analysis of clinical studies. Clin Immunol 2010;137(1):21–30.

25. Lucas M, Lee M, Lortan J, et al. Infection outcomes in patients with common variable immunodeficiency disorders: relationship to immunoglobulin therapy over 22 years. J Allergy Clin Immunol 2010;125(6):1354–1360 e4.

26. Shapiro RS, Wasserman RL, Bonagura V, et al. Emerging Paradigm of Primary Immunodeficiency Disease: Individualizing Immunoglobulin Dose and Delivery to Enhance Outcomes. J Clin Immunol 2017;37(2):190–6.

27. Bonilla FA. Intravenous immunoglobulin: adverse reactions and management. J Allergy Clin Immunol 2008;122(6):1238–9.

28. Hajjar J, Kutac C, Rider NL, et al. Fatigue and the wear-off effect in adult patients with common variable immunodeficiency. Clin Exp Immunol 2018;194(3):327–38.

29. Rojavin MA, Hubsch A, Lawo JP. Quantitative Evidence of Wear-Off Effect at the End of the Intravenous IgG (IVIG) Dosing Cycle in Primary Immunodeficiency. J Clin Immunol 2016;36(3):210–9.

30. Quartier P, Debre M, De Blic J, et al. Early and prolonged intravenous immunoglobulin replacement therapy in childhood agammaglobulinemia: a retrospective survey of 31 patients. J Pediatr 1999;134(5):589–96.

31. Rigante D, Frediani B, Cantarini L. A Comprehensive Overview of the Hereditary Periodic Fever Syndromes. Clin Rev Allergy Immunol 2018;54(3):446–53.

32. Ferre EMN, Schmitt MM, Lionakis MS. Autoimmune Polyendocrinopathy-Candidiasis-Ectodermal Dystrophy. Front Pediatr 2021;9:723532.

33. Barzaghi F, Amaya Hernandez LC, Neven B, et al. Long-term follow-up of IPEX syndrome patients after different therapeutic strategies: An international multicenter retrospective study. J Allergy Clin Immunol 2018;141(3):1036–49, e5.

34. Rao VK, Oliveira JB. How I treat autoimmune lymphoproliferative syndrome. Blood 2011;118(22):5741–51.

35. Dorsey MJ, Wright NAM, Chaimowitz NS, et al. Infections in Infants with SCID: Isolation, Infection Screening, and Prophylaxis in PIDTC Centers. J Clin Immunol 2021;41(1):38–50.

36. Heimall J, Logan BR, Cowan MJ, et al. Immune reconstitution and survival of 100 SCID patients post-hematopoietic cell transplant: a PIDTC natural history study. Blood 2017;130(25):2718–27.

37. Buckley RH. Transplantation of hematopoietic stem cells in human severe combined immunodeficiency: longterm outcomes. Immunol Res 2011;49(1–3):25–43.

38. Haddad E, Logan BR, Griffith LM, et al. SCID genotype and 6-month posttransplant CD4 count predict survival and immune recovery. Blood 2018;132(17):1737–49.
39. Al-Mofareh M, Ayas M, Al-Seraihy A, et al. Hematopoietic stem cell transplantation in children with Griscelli syndrome type 2: a single-center report on 35 patients. Bone Marrow Transpl 2020;55(10):2026–34.
40. Huizing M, Malicdan MCV, Gochuico BR, Gahl WA. Hermansky-Pudlak Syndrome. 2000. [updated 2021 Mar 18], In: Adam MP, Everman DB, Mirzaa GM, et al. GeneReviews® [Internet], Seattle (WA): University of Washington, Seattle, 1993–2022.
41. Toro C., Nicoli E.R., Malicdan M.C., et al., Chediak-Higashi Syndrome. 2009. [updated 2018 Jul 5]. In: Adam M.P., Everman D.B., Mirzaa G.M., et al., editors. GeneReviews® [Internet]. Seattle (WA): University of Washington, Seattle; 1993–2022.
42. Kuo CY, Kohn DB. Overview of the current status of gene therapy for primary immune deficiencies (PIDs). J Allergy Clin Immunol 2020;146(2):229–33.
43. Fischer A, Notarangelo LD, Neven B, et al. Severe combined immunodeficiencies and related disorders. Nat Rev Dis Primers 2015;1:15061.
44. Davies EG, Cheung M, Gilmour K, et al. Thymus transplantation for complete DiGeorge syndrome: European experience. J Allergy Clin Immunol 2017;140(6):1660–1670 e16.
45. Giardino G, Radwan N, Koletsi P, et al. Clinical and immunological features in a cohort of patients with partial DiGeorge syndrome followed at a single center. Blood 2019;133(24):2586–96.
46. Markert ML, Gupton SE, McCarthy EA. Experience with cultured thymus tissue in 105 children. J Allergy Clin Immunol 2022;149(2):747–57.
47. Buchbinder D, Nugent DJ, Fillipovich AH. Wiskott-Aldrich syndrome: diagnosis, current management, and emerging treatments. Appl Clin Genet 2014;7:55–66.
48. Candotti F. Clinical manifestations and pathophysiological mechanisms of the wiskott-aldrich syndrome. J Clin Immunol 2018;38(1):13–27.
49. Leven EA, Maffucci P, Ochs HD, et al. Hyper IgM syndrome: a report from the USIDNET registry. J Clin Immunol 2016;36(5):490–501.
50. Amirifar P, Ranjouri MR, Lavin M, et al. Ataxia-telangiectasia: epidemiology, pathogenesis, clinical phenotype, diagnosis, prognosis and management. Expert Rev Clin Immunol 2020;16(9):859–71.
51. Mogensen TH. STAT3 and the Hyper-IgE syndrome: Clinical presentation, genetic origin, pathogenesis, novel findings and remaining uncertainties. JAKSTAT 2013;2(2):e23435.
52. Cunningham-Rundles C. The many faces of common variable immunodeficiency. Hematol Am Soc Hematol Educ Program 2012;2012:301–5.
53. Winkelstein JA, Marino MC, Lederman HM, et al. X-linked agammaglobulinemia: report on a United States registry of 201 patients. Medicine (Baltimore) 2006;85(4):193–202.
54. Aghamohammadi A, Mohammadi J, Parvaneh N, et al. Progression of selective IgA deficiency to common variable immunodeficiency. Int Arch Allergy Immunol 2008;147(2):87–92.
55. Yel L. Selective IgA deficiency. J Clin Immunol 2010;30(1):10–6.
56. Qamar N, Fuleihan RL. The hyper IgM syndromes. Clin Rev Allergy Immunol 2014;46(2):120–30.
57. Sorensen RU, Edgar D. Specific antibody deficiencies in clinical practice. J Allergy Clin Immunol Pract 2019;7(3):801–8.

58. Stiehm ER. The four most common pediatric immunodeficiencies. J Immunotoxicol 2008;5(2):227–34.
59. Chiriaco M, Salfa I, Di Matteo G, et al. Chronic granulomatous disease: Clinical, molecular, and therapeutic aspects. Pediatr Allergy Immunol 2016;27(3):242–53.
60. Thomsen IP, Smith MA, Holland SM, et al. A comprehensive approach to the management of children and adults with chronic granulomatous disease. J Allergy Clin Immunol Pract 2016;4(6):1082–8.
61. Hanna S, Etzioni A. Leukocyte adhesion deficiencies. Ann N Y Acad Sci 2012; 1250:50–5.
62. Hsu AP, McReynolds LJ, Holland SM. GATA2 deficiency. Curr Opin Allergy Clin Immunol 2015;15(1):104–9.
63. Wen L, Atkinson JP, Giclas PC. Clinical and laboratory evaluation of complement deficiency. J Allergy Clin Immunol 2004;113(4):585–93 [quiz: 594].
64. Price S, Shaw PA, Seitz A, et al. Natural history of autoimmune lymphoproliferative syndrome associated with FAS gene mutations. Blood 2014;123(13):1989–99.
65. Ferre EM, Rose SR, Rosenzweig SD, et al. Redefined clinical features and diagnostic criteria in autoimmune polyendocrinopathy-candidiasis-ectodermal dystrophy. JCI Insight 2016;1(13). https://doi.org/10.1172/jci.insight.88782.
66. Wildin RS, Smyk-Pearson S, Filipovich AH. Clinical and molecular features of the immunodysregulation, polyendocrinopathy, enteropathy, X linked (IPEX) syndrome. J Med Genet 2002;39(8):537–45.
67. Booshehri LM, Hoffman HM. CAPS and NLRP3. J Clin Immunol 2019;39(3): 277–86.

Oral Immunotherapy
An Overview

Krista Todoric, MD[a],*, Sarah Merrill, MD[b]

KEYWORDS

- Oral immunotherapy • OIT • Food allergy • Tolerance
- Sustained unresponsiveness • Peanut • Milk • Egg

KEY POINTS

- Avoidance has historically been the sole treatment option for Immunoglobulin E (IgE)-mediated food allergy, although oral immunotherapy (OIT) is now an alternative approach.
- OIT effects may be dependent on dose, duration, and frequency of dosing as well as patient-specific factors, such as age and food-specific IgE levels.
- There is only one U.S. Food and Drug Administration (FDA)-approved OIT product (Palforzia, for peanut); otherwise, OIT occurs through the use of commercially available food products.
- Multifood OIT protocols seem to be as safe as single-food protocols, and biological therapies may assist with tolerability of OIT protocols and further improve success rates.
- Studies to date looking at sustained unresponsiveness and remission suggest that OIT needs to be continued in some manner for most individuals to have persistent effects.

INTRODUCTION

The prevalence of IgE-mediated food allergy (FA) continues to increase across the globe, with rates as high as 9% in children and 4% in adults[1-5] and a noted 50% increase in the United States from 1999 to 2011.[1,2,6] Despite decades of research, there is no known cure for FA,[6] and strict dietary elimination and food avoidance have been the basis of treatment.[7] Given the ubiquitous presence of the most common allergenic foods, avoidance is challenging, and accidental ingestions are seen frequently[1]; nearly 40% of the estimated 5.9 million FA children in the United States have experienced a severe life-threatening reaction.[8] Both financial and social costs in FA are also high. The economic impact of pediatric FA in the United States amounts to US$4.3 billion annually in direct medical costs,[3,9] and studies show negative quality of life indicators for both patients and caregivers,[10] with 50% of FA children experiencing bullying.[6]

[a] Medical Arts Allergy, 220 Wilson Street Suite 200, Carlisle, PA 17013, USA; [b] Family Medicine Department, UC San Diego Health, 402 Dickinson Street, San Diego, CA 92103, USA
* Corresponding author.
E-mail address: ktodorich@gmail.com

Prim Care Clin Office Pract 50 (2023) 269–281
https://doi.org/10.1016/j.pop.2022.11.006
primarycare.theclinics.com
0095-4543/23/© 2022 Elsevier Inc. All rights reserved.

More recently, oral immunotherapy (OIT) has emerged as a promising alternative treatment strategy in FA. OIT is a program of supervised swallowed food introduction, typically involving 1 day of desensitization, multiple-dose escalation visits, and maintenance dosing thereafter (**Fig. 1**). The primary goal of OIT in clinical practice is protection against accidental exposure to an allergen triggering anaphylaxis. Some patients will reach an amount of food ingestion that, secondarily, allows them to incorporate the food unrestrictedly into their diet. Although OIT should be pursued only under the direction of an allergist, it is important for primary care physicians who diagnose, guide appropriate referral to specialty care, and are likely to also participate in the care of increasing numbers of individuals choosing OIT as an FA treatment strategy to be aware of this novel approach to FA.

OIT is not without the risk of adverse reactions (ARs). Most ARs occur during dose escalation (but may occur at any time during OIT) and most commonly include self-limited or antihistamine-treated oropharyngeal pruritus or transient abdominal pain.[11] At times, these early symptoms may require extensive protocol adjustment. Not insignificantly, up to 10% of OIT patients can exhibit respiratory symptoms,[7] and an estimated 10% to 15% of patients withdrew from studies due to severe, intolerable abdominal pain.[7,11] Frequency of anaphylaxis and epinephrine use among OIT patients is generally increased compared to the those practicing food avoidance.[12] Eosinophilic esophagitis has also been postulated as a complication of OIT treatment, although it is unclear if this is present before or resulting from OIT.[11,13] Factors increasing the risk of ARs include concurrent illness, physical exertion following dose administration, menstruation, poorly controlled asthma, and timing with food ingestion.[11] OIT-dosing guidances are advised to diminish the risk of ARs but can affect lifestyle and be challenging in individuals of varying age and taste preference. As such, size, formulation, and frequency of OIT doses as well as coadministration of biological therapies to improve tolerability remain current hot topics in OIT research.

Oral tolerance is the state of unresponsiveness to an antigen. Desensitization is an increase in reaction threshold to a food allergen while receiving active therapy such as OIT. Sustained unresponsiveness (SU) is the safe reintroduction of a food after a period of avoidance, often used as a surrogate marker for more permanent clinical unresponsiveness after OIT. Remission has been used more recently to describe those with longer term SU. Use of biomarker profiles and commercially available tests, such as basophil activation testing[14] and bead-based epitope assay,[15] to more reliably predict clinical tolerance threshold and those who will maintain SU or enter remission

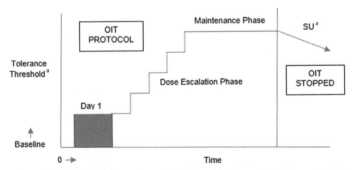

Fig. 1. Overview of OIT protocol and results. [a]May be dependent on age, dose, duration, frequency of dosing, among others.

show promise but require further investigation and validation for consistent application in clinical practice and OIT.

DISCUSSION
Peanut Oral Immunotherapy

Peanut has been one of the most studied foods used in OIT and is the only food for which there is a current FDA-approved OIT product (Palforzia). Several randomized trials[16–29] and several uncontrolled studies[30–38] have demonstrated that peanut OIT (POIT) is highly effective at inducing desensitization and increasing tolerance threshold, up to 2 to 18 times the maintenance dose,[18–20,25,27,28,30,32,35,37–40] although this may be dependent on duration[41] and frequency of dosing.[42] A systematic review of 12 trials with 1041 patients showed that POIT increased the likelihood of passing an in-clinic supervised food challenge (relative risk [RR] 12.42) but also increased anaphylaxis risk (RR 3.12), anaphylaxis frequency (incidence rate ratio 2.72), and epinephrine use (RR 2.21) compared with those strictly avoiding peanut.[42] SU is much less common and may be dependent on dose and duration as well as dependent on the age of the individual when POIT is initiated and certain biomarker parameters (such as food-specific IgE).[16,22,31,38,42,43,44] Only 2 studies have evaluated longer term SU, or remission, and both noted a decreasing tolerance threshold effect with increased time from POIT end,[22,44] although this remained higher than baseline and different from those who never started POIT.[44] Lower baseline peanut-specific IgE and younger age at screening predicted remission.[22]

Milk Oral Immunotherapy

To date, milk OIT (MOIT) has only been studied in children to a typical target maintenance dose of 100 to 250 mL milk, and desensitization was achieved in 36% to 97%.[45–60] Low-dose (0.5–10 mL) milk with escalation to 150 to 200 mL has demonstrated high rates of desensitization (98%) when started in infants aged younger than 1 year,[54,61,62] and longer term lower dose MOIT can also increase tolerance threshold[63] and rates of desensitization[64,65] as well as induce SU.[66,67] Meta-analysis of 5 MOIT trials with 218 children showed that MOIT increased the likelihood of developing full tolerance to milk by 10-fold but also increased the risk of AR by 34-fold, with an RR of 5.8 for needing epinephrine.[68] Fewer studies have evaluated SU in MOIT, with rates varying from 25.6%[49] to 40%[57] and increasing with longer duration of MOIT.[49]

Roughly 70% of patient with cow's milk allergy may tolerate baked milk (BM), and tolerating BM may accelerate the resolution of cow's milk allergy.[69–72] Formalized introduction of baked milk OIT (BMOIT) can significantly increase tolerance threshold[73] and time to desensitization to unbaked milk compared with controls.[72–74] In addition, one study noted no difference in rates of desensitization or daily dose of cow's milk being consumed at end of study between those treated with BMOIT or MOIT, although there was a significant trend to increased adverse events in the BMOIT group.[59]

Egg Oral Immunotherapy

Egg OIT (EOIT) has been evaluated in children in several controlled[75–84] and uncontrolled studies[85–90] with rates of desensitization ranging from 36% to 94%[79,82,91–93] and increase in tolerance threshold by 2 to 10-fold,[81,94] likely dependent on age,[81] protocol design,[83] maintenance dosing regimens,[84] and duration of therapy.[83,95] A Cochrane review performed in 2018 that included 10 RCTs with 439 children aged from 1 to 18 years showed EOIT increased tolerance threshold to egg and complete recovery from allergy compared with controls.[96] Those studies looking at SU show higher rates in those treated with EOIT compared with avoidance[75,78,88,96,97] and in those on longer duration of therapy.[78]

Tolerance of baked egg (BE) may occur before tolerance to unbaked egg,[98] and early BE introduction, even at low dose, can decrease the rate of unbaked egg allergy.[99] Baked egg OIT (BEOIT) can desensitize and increase tolerance threshold to unbaked egg in BE-intolerant children, although these effects may be dependent on dose and duration and have not been rigorously evaluated against a control population.[89,90,100,101] One study looking at low-dose BEOIT has demonstrated increased rates of desensitization and SU to unbaked egg compared with controls.[88] Only one study has compared outcomes in 55 children aged 3 to 16 years tolerant to BE who continue BE ingestion or completed a course of EOIT.[102] In this study, the EOIT group had better outcomes at the year 1 and 2 food challenges compared with the BE group ($P = .002$ and $P < .0001$, respectively) and significantly more of the EOIT group achieved 8 to 10 week SU compared with the BE group (43.5% vs 11.1%, $P = .009$).[102]

Wheat Oral Immunotherapy

Six small pilot studies[103–108] and one controlled trial[109] of wheat OIT (WOIT) in children reported 85% to 100% desensitization with a wide range of maintenance doses (400–70,000 mg) during 3 to 24 months, although these effects may be dependent on dose and duration.[109–111] Fewer studies have evaluated SU in WOIT,[109,111] with increasing rates of 2 week SU with increased duration of WOIT[111,112] even when low-dose (53 mg) WOIT is used.[111]

Sesame Oral Immunotherapy

One study with sesame OIT showed that 88.3% achieved full desensitization to 4000 mg sesame at end of dose escalation, and 100% of these individuals maintained 4000 mg desensitization even with maintenance dose reduction to 1200 mg for at least 6 months (compared with no controls).[113]

Tree Nut Oral Immunotherapy

One controlled study[114,115] and one retrospective[116] study evaluated tree nut OIT (TNOIT). These have shown that walnut, cashew, and hazelnut OIT can induce desensitization and increase tolerance thresholds,[114–116] with possible increase with longer duration of therapy.[116] Additionally, walnut and cashew OIT can desensitize to coallergic tree nuts.[114,115] After walnut-specific TNOIT, 100% pecan, 93% hazelnut, and 60% hazelnut or cashew coallergic individuals were desensitized to the coallergic nut(s).[115] Following cashew-specific TNOIT, 100% pistachio and 50% walnut coallergic patients were desensitized to their coallergic nut(s).[114]

Multifood Oral Immunotherapy

There has been one randomized trial evaluating the safety and efficacy of multifood OIT as a sole therapeutic intervention compared with single food OIT.[117] In this study, up to 5 food allergens could be used with dose escalation to 4000 mg protein of each allergen.[117] Time to reach 300, 1000, 4000 mg, and a 10-fold increase in threshold dose were significantly longer in the multifood OIT group compared with the single food OIT group ($P \leq .005$).[117] Rates of reaction per dose did not differ significantly between the 2 groups ($P = .31$).[117]

Other Considerations

Modified food sources, adjuvants, and coadministration of other therapies to improve OIT outcomes have been evaluated. Extensively hydrolyzed MOIT and EOIT did not desensitize to intact protein,[77,118] although *partially* hydrolyzed milk and wheat OIT[119] did improve tolerance threshold. Peanut plus probiotic OIT subjects achieved desensitization, although there was no comparison with POIT alone.[120] A preclinical study in mice showed that nanoparticles containing peanut protected from anaphylaxis.[121]

Coadministration of etokimab (IL33 antagonist) and omalizumab (IgE antagonist) improved tolerance threshold in OIT patients,[122,123] and omalizumab has also decreased food reactions and improved safety in OIT.[123] There are 3 current studies underway to evaluate the effectiveness of omalizumab in multifood OIT, alone[124–126] and in combination with a Chinese herbal.[127] There are 3 planned studies looking at dupilumab (IL4/13 antagonist), the first to evaluate if its concomitant use increases the proportion of individuals on Palforzia OIT who pass a challenge at 4 months[128] and the second to evaluate if peanut-allergic individuals can achieve full tolerance without OIT.[129] A third study will evaluate whether omalizumab plus dupilumab will act synergistically to improve tolerance to 2 or more foods compared with omalizumab alone.[130]

SUMMARY

OIT is an alternative treatment of IgE-mediated FA that has been shown to increase tolerance threshold to many of the top food allergens, although this effect may be dependent on age, dose, frequency, and duration. OIT has been shown to be effective and safe in infants, and early initiation can improve rates of desensitization even for those foods whose natural history favors loss of allergy. Studies looking at protocol modification to improve OIT success are ongoing as is the evaluation of clinical tools to help monitor OIT effects.

CLINICS CARE POINTS

- IgE-mediated FA prevalence is increasing across the globe, with no known cure. Avoidance has been the historically sole treatment option.
- OIT is now an alternative treatment of IgE-mediated FA.
- OIT effects may be dependent on dose, duration, and frequency of dosing as well as patient-specific factors, such as age and food-specific IgE levels.
- There is only one FDA-approved OIT product (Palforzia, for peanut); otherwise, OIT occurs through use of commercially available food products.
- Multifood OIT protocols seem to be as safe as single-food protocols.
- Biological therapies may assist with tolerability of OIT protocols and further improve success rates.
- Studies to date looking at SU and remission suggest that OIT will need to be continued in some manner for most individuals for persistence of effects.
- Individuals who present with shortness of breath, wheezing, coughing, hives, nausea/vomiting, swelling, and loss of consciousness following food ingestion should be evaluated for the potential of IgE-mediated FA. If diagnosed, they should also be counseled on the availability of OIT as a treatment option and referred to an allergist for comanagement.

- When a patient experiences systemic symptoms while undergoing OIT therapy, these symptoms should be treated as with any other accidental ingestion, including the use of epinephrine if warranted.
- If systemic symptoms are experienced during OIT, a detailed history is required to evaluate for modifiable cofactors that can influence OIT dose reactivity, such as concurrent illness, exercise/activities surrounding timing of dose, food ingestions, menstruation, and oral sores, among others.
- Onset of abdominal pain and nausea/vomiting after initiation of OIT should prompt the evaluation for OIT-adverse effects, such as eosinophilic esophagitis, which may necessitate cessation of OIT therapy.
- If OIT protocol deviations are encountered and doses are missed, patients are at risk of systemic reaction with reinitiation of dosing, and dosing should only be restarted under the guidance of an allergist experienced in OIT.

DISCLOSURE

The authors have nothing to disclose.

REFERENCES

1. Egan M, Greenhawt M. Common questions in food allergy avoidance. Ann Allergy Asthma Immunol 2018;120:263–71.
2. Feng C. Beyond Avoidance: the Psychosocial Impact of Food Allergies. Clin Rev Allergy Immunol 2019;57:74–82.
3. Dyer A, Negris O, Gupta R, et al. Food allergy: how expensive are they? Curr Opin Allergy Immunol 2020;20(2):188–93.
4. Shaker M, Greenhawt M. Providing cost-effective care for food allergy. Ann Allergy Asthma Immunol 2019;123(3):240–8.
5. Cerecedo I, Zamora J, Fox M, et al. The impact of double-blind placebo-controlled food challenge (DBPCFC) on the socioeconomic cost of food allergy in Europe. J Investig Allergol Clin Immunol 2014;24(6):418–24.
6. Peters R, Krawiec M, Koplin J, et al. Update on food allergy. Pediatr Allergy Immunol 2021;32:647–57.
7. Mori F, Cianferoni A, Brambilla A, et al. Side effects and their impact on the success of milk oral immunotherapy in children. Int J Immunopathology Pharmacol 2017;32(2):182–7.
8. Bilaver L, Kester K, Smith B, et al. Socioeconomic disparities in the economic impact of childhood food allergy. Pediatrics 2016;137(5):e20153678.
9. Gupta R, Holdford D, Bilaver L, et al. The economic impact of childhood food allergy in the United States. JAMA Pediatr 2013;167(11):1026–31.
10. Golding M, Batac A, Gunnarsson N, et al. The burden of food allergy on children and teens: A systematic review. Pediatr Allergy Immunol 2022;33(3):e13743.
11. Scurlock A. Oral and sublingual immunotherapy for treatment of ige-mediated food allergy. Clin Rev Allergy Immunol 2018;55:139–52.
12. Chu DK, Wood RA, French S, et al. Oral immunotherapy for peanut allergy (PACE): a systematic review and meta-analysis of efficacy and safety. Lancet 2019;393(10187):2222–32.
13. Jin H, Trogen B, Nowak-Wergrzyn A. Eosinophilic esophagitis as a complication of food oral immunotherapy. Curr Opin Allergy Clin Immunol 2020;20(6):616–23.

14. Santos AF, Alpan O, Hoffmann HJ. Basophil activation test: Mechanisms and considerations for use in clinical trials and clinical practice. Allergy 2021; 76(8):2420–32.

15. Suprun M, Getts R, Raghunathan R, et al. Novel Bead-Based Epitope Assay is a sensitive and reliable tool for profiling epitope-specific antibody repertoire in food allergy. Sci Rep 2019;9(1):18425.

16. Vickery BP, Berglund JP, Burk CM, et al. Early oral immunotherapy in peanut-allergic preschool children is safe and highly effective. J Allergy Clin Immunol 2017;139(1):173–81, e8.

17. Varshney P, Jones SM, Scurlock AM, et al. A randomized controlled study of peanut oral immunotherapy: clinical desensitization and modulation of the allergic response. J Allergy Clin Immunol 2011;127(3):654–60.

18. Anagnostou K, Islam S, King Y, et al. Assessing the efficacy of oral immunotherapy for the desensitisation of peanut allergy in children (STOP II): a phase 2 randomised controlled trial. Lancet 2014;383(9925):1297–304.

19. Bird JA, Spergel JM, Jones SM, et al. Efficacy and safety of AR101 in oral immunotherapy for peanut allergy: results of ARC001, a randomized, double-blind, placebo-controlled phase 2 clinical trial. J Allergy Clin Immunol Pract 2018; 6(2):476–85, e3.

20. Vickery BP, Vereda A, Casale TB, et al. AR101 oral immunotherapy for peanut allergy. N Engl J Med 2018;379(21):1991–2001.

21. Reier-Nilsen T, Michelsen MM, Lødrup Carlsen KC, et al. Feasibility of desensitizing children highly allergic to peanut by high-dose oral immunotherapy. Allergy 2019;74(2):337–48.

22. Jones SM, Kim EH, Nadeau KC, et al. Efficacy and safety of oral immunotherapy in children aged 1-3 years with peanut allergy (the Immune Tolerance Network IMPACT trial): a randomised placebo-controlled study. Lancet 2022;399(10322): 359–71.

23. Nagakura KI, Sato S, Yanagida N, et al. Oral immunotherapy in japanese children with anaphylactic peanut allergy. Int Arch Allergy Immunol 2018;175(3): 181–8.

24. Anvari S, Tran D, Nguyen A, et al. Peanut oral immunotherapy dose variations do not result in allergic reactions. Pediatr Allergy Immunol 2018;29(2):218–20.

25. Kukkonen AK, Uotila R, Malmberg LP, et al. Double-blind placebo-controlled challenge showed that peanut oral immunotherapy was effective for severe allergy without negative effects on airway inflammation. Acta Paediatr 2017; 106(2):274–81.

26. Fauquert JL, Michaud E, Pereira B, et al. Peanut gastrointestinal delivery oral immunotherapy in adolescents: Results of the build-up phase of a randomized, double-blind, placebo-controlled trial (PITA study). Clin Exp Allergy 2018;48(7): 862–74.

27. Bluemchen K, Eiwegger T. Oral peanut immunotherapy How much is too much? How much is enough? Allergy 2019;74(2):220–2.

28. Narisety SD, Frischmeyer-Guerrerio PA, Keet CA, et al. A randomized, double-blind, placebo-controlled pilot study of sublingual versus oral immunotherapy for the treatment of peanut allergy. J Allergy Clin Immunol 2015;135(5): 1275–82, e1-6.

29. O'B Hourihane J, Beyer K, Abbas A, et al. Efficacy and safety of oral immunotherapy with AR101 in European children with a peanut allergy (ARTEMIS): a multicentre, double-blind, randomised, placebo-controlled phase 3 trial. Lancet Child Adolesc Health 2020;4(10):728–39.

30. Anagnostou K, Clark A, King Y, et al. Efficacy and safety of high-dose peanut oral immunotherapy with factors predicting outcome. Clin Exp Allergy 2011; 41(9):1273–81.

31. Vickery BP, Scurlock AM, Kulis M, et al. Sustained unresponsiveness to peanut in subjects who have completed peanut oral immunotherapy. J Allergy Clin Immunol 2014;133(2):468–75.

32. Jones SM, Pons L, Roberts JL, et al. Clinical efficacy and immune regulation with peanut oral immunotherapy. J Allergy Clin Immunol 2009;124(2):292–300, e1-97.

33. Nurmatov U, Venderbosch I, Devereux G, et al. Allergen-specific oral immunotherapy for peanut allergy. Cochrane Database Syst Rev 2012;9:CD009014.

34. Burks AW, Laubach S, Jones SM. Oral tolerance, food allergy, and immunotherapy: implications for future treatment. J Allergy Clin Immunol 2008;121(6): 1344–50.

35. Blumchen K, Ulbricht H, Staden U, et al. Oral peanut immunotherapy in children with peanut anaphylaxis. J Allergy Clin Immunol 2010;126(1):83–91.e1.

36. Nachshon L, Goldberg MR, Katz Y, et al. Long-term outcome of peanut oral immunotherapy-Real-life experience. Pediatr Allergy Immunol 2018;29(5): 519–26.

37. Nagakura KI, Yanagida N, Sato S, et al. Low-dose oral immunotherapy for children with anaphylactic peanut allergy in Japan. Pediatr Allergy Immunol 2018; 29(5):512–8.

38. Wasserman RL, Hague AR, Pence DM, et al. Real-world experience with peanut oral immunotherapy: lessons learned from 270 patients. J Allergy Clin Immunol Pract 2019;7(2):418–26, e4.

39. Zhong Y, Chew JL, Tan MM, et al. Efficacy and safety of oral immunotherapy for peanut allergy: a pilot study in Singaporean children. Asia Pac Allergy 2019; 9(1):e1.

40. Bird JA, Feldman M, Arneson A, et al. Modified peanut oral immunotherapy protocol safely and effectively induces desensitization. J Allergy Clin Immunol Pract 2015;3(3):433–5, e1-3.

41. Fernandez-Rivas M, Vereda A, Vickery BP, et al. Open-label follow-on study evaluating the efficacy, safety, and quality of life with extended daily oral immunotherapy in children with peanut allergy. Allergy 2022;77(3):991–1003.

42. Vickery BP, Vereda A, Nilsson C, et al. Continuous and daily oral immunotherapy for peanut allergy: results from a 2-year open-label follow-on study. J Allergy Clin Immunol Pract 2021;9(5):1879–89, e14.

43. Herlihy L, Kim EH, Burks AW, et al. Five-year follow-up of early intervention peanut oral immunotherapy. J Allergy Clin Immunol Pract 2021;9(1):514–7.

44. Chinthrajah RS, Purington N, Andorf S, et al. Sustained outcomes in oral immunotherapy for peanut allergy (POISED study): a large, randomised, double-blind, placebo-controlled, phase 2 study. Lancet 2019;394(10207):1437–49.

45. Meglio P, Bartone E, Plantamura M, et al. A protocol for oral desensitization in children with IgE-mediated cow's milk allergy. Allergy 2004;59(9):980–7.

46. Longo G, Barbi E, Berti I, et al. Specific oral tolerance induction in children with very severe cow's milk-induced reactions. J Allergy Clin Immunol 2008;121(2): 343–7.

47. Pajno GB. Oral desensitization for milk allergy in children: state of the art. Curr Opin Allergy Clin Immunol 2011;11(6):560–4.

48. Martorell A, De la Hoz B, Ibáñez MD, et al. Oral desensitization as a useful treatment in 2-year-old children with cow's milk allergy. Clin Exp Allergy 2011;41(9): 1297–304.

49. Takahashi M, Taniuchi S, Soejima K, et al. Two-weeks-sustained unresponsiveness by oral immunotherapy using microwave heated cow's milk for children with cow's milk allergy. Allergy Asthma Clin Immunol 2016;12(1):44.

50. Ebrahimi M, Gharagozlou M, Mohebbi A, et al. The efficacy of oral immunotherapy in patients with cow's milk allergy. Iran J Allergy Asthma Immunol 2017;16(3):183–92.

51. Mota I, Piedade S, Gaspar Â, et al. Cow's milk oral immunotherapy in real life: 8-year long-term follow-up study. Asia Pac Allergy 2018;8(3):e28.

52. Kauppila TK, Paassilta M, Kukkonen AK, et al. Outcome of oral immunotherapy for persistent cow's milk allergy from 11 years of experience in Finland. Pediatr Allergy Immunol 2019;30(3):356–62.

53. De Schryver S, Mazer B, Clarke AE, et al. Adverse events in oral immunotherapy for the desensitization of cow's milk allergy in children: a randomized controlled trial. J Allergy Clin Immunol Pract 2019;7(6):1912–9.

54. Berti I, Badina L, Cozzi G, et al. Early oral immunotherapy in infants with cow's milk protein allergy. Pediatr Allergy Immunol 2019;30(5):572–4.

55. Vázquez-Ortiz M, Alvaro-Lozano M, Alsina L, et al. Safety and predictors of adverse events during oral immunotherapy for milk allergy: severity of reaction at oral challenge, specific IgE and prick test. Clin Exp Allergy 2013;43(1): 92–102.

56. Levy MB, Elizur A, Goldberg MR, et al. Clinical predictors for favorable outcomes in an oral immunotherapy program for IgE-mediated cow's milk allergy. Ann Allergy Asthma Immunol 2014;112(1):58–63.e1.

57. Keet CA, Frischmeyer-Guerrerio PA, Thyagarajan A, et al. The safety and efficacy of sublingual and oral immunotherapy for milk allergy. J Allergy Clin Immunol 2012;129(2):448–55, 55.e1-5.

58. Perezábad L, Reche M, Valbuena T, et al. Oral food desensitization in children with ige-mediated cow's milk allergy: immunological changes underlying desensitization. Allergy Asthma Immunol Res 2017;9(1):35–42.

59. Amat F, Kouche C, Gaspard W, et al. Is a slow-progression baked milk protocol of oral immunotherapy always a safe option for children with cow's milk allergy? A randomized controlled trial. Clin Exp Allergy 2017;47(11):1491–6.

60. Yeung JP, Kloda LA, McDevitt J, et al. Oral immunotherapy for milk allergy. Cochrane Database Syst Rev 2012;11:CD009542.

61. Badina L, Levantino L, Carrato V, et al. Early introduction oral immunotherapy for IgE-mediated cow's milk allergy: A follow-up study confirms this approach as safe and appealing to parents. Immun Inflamm Dis 2021;9(3):918–22.

62. Boné Calvo J, Clavero Adell M, Guallar Abadía I, et al. As soon as possible in IgE-cow's milk allergy immunotherapy. Eur J Pediatr 2021;180(1):291–4.

63. Takaoka Y, Yajima Y, Ito YM, et al. Single-Center Noninferiority Randomized Trial on the Efficacy and Safety of Low- and High-Dose Rush Oral Milk Immunotherapy for Severe Milk Allergy. Int Arch Allergy Immunol 2020;181(9):699–705.

64. Skripak JM, Nash SD, Rowley H, et al. A randomized, double-blind, placebo-controlled study of milk oral immunotherapy for cow's milk allergy. J Allergy Clin Immunol 2008;122(6):1154–60.

65. Narisety SD, Skripak JM, Steele P, et al. Open-label maintenance after milk oral immunotherapy for IgE-mediated cow's milk allergy. J Allergy Clin Immunol 2009;124(3):610–2.

66. Yanagida N, Sato S, Asaumi T, et al. A Single-Center, Case-Control Study of Low-Dose-Induction Oral Immunotherapy with Cow's Milk. Int Arch Allergy Immunol 2015;168(2):131–7.

67. Miura Y, Nagakura KI, Nishino M, et al. Long-term follow-up of fixed low-dose oral immunotherapy for children with severe cow's milk allergy. Pediatr Allergy Immunol 2021;32(4):734–41.

68. Brożek JL, Terracciano L, Hsu J, et al. Oral immunotherapy for IgE-mediated cow's milk allergy: a systematic review and meta-analysis. Clin Exp Allergy 2012;42(3):363–74.

69. Luyt D, Ball H, Makwana N, et al. BSACI guideline for the diagnosis and management of cow's milk allergy. Clin Exp Allergy 2014;44(5):642–72.

70. Kim JS, Nowak-Węgrzyn A, Sicherer SH, et al. Dietary baked milk accelerates the resolution of cow's milk allergy in children. J Allergy Clin Immunol 2011; 128(1):125–31.e2.

71. Nowak-Węgrzyn A, Sampson HA. Future therapies for food allergies. J Allergy Clin Immunol 2011;127(3):558–73, quiz 74-5.

72. Esmaeilzadeh H, Alyasin S, Haghighat M, et al. The effect of baked milk on accelerating unheated cow's milk tolerance: A control randomized clinical trial. Pediatr Allergy Immunol 2018;29(7):747–53.

73. Goldberg MR, Nachshon L, Appel MY, et al. Efficacy of baked milk oral immunotherapy in baked milk-reactive allergic patients. J Allergy Clin Immunol 2015;136(6):1601–6.

74. Efron A, Zeldin Y, Gotesdyner L, et al. A structured gradual exposure protocol to baked and heated milk in the treatment of milk allergy. J Pediatr 2018;203: 204–9.e2.

75. Burks AW, Jones SM, Wood RA, et al. Oral immunotherapy for treatment of egg allergy in children. N Engl J Med 2012;367(3):233–43.

76. Escudero C, Rodríguez Del Río P, Sánchez-García S, et al. Early sustained unresponsiveness after short-course egg oral immunotherapy: a randomized controlled study in egg-allergic children. Clin Exp Allergy 2015;45(12):1833–43.

77. Giavi S, Vissers YM, Muraro A, et al. Oral immunotherapy with low allergenic hydrolysed egg in egg allergic children. Allergy 2016;71(11):1575–84.

78. Jones SM, Burks AW, Keet C, et al. Long-term treatment with egg oral immunotherapy enhances sustained unresponsiveness that persists after cessation of therapy. J Allergy Clin Immunol 2016;137(4):1117–27, e10.

79. Pérez-Rangel I, Rodríguez Del Río P, Escudero C, et al. Efficacy and safety of high-dose rush oral immunotherapy in persistent egg allergic children: A randomized clinical trial. Ann Allergy Asthma Immunol 2017;118(3):356–64, e3.

80. Takaoka Y, Maeta A, Takahashi K, et al. Effectiveness and safety of double-blind, placebo-controlled, low-dose oral immunotherapy with low allergen egg-containing cookies for severe hen's egg allergy: a single-center analysis. Int Arch Allergy Immunol 2019;180(4):244–9.

81. Itoh-Nagato N, Inoue Y, Nagao M, et al. Desensitization to a whole egg by rush oral immunotherapy improves the quality of life of guardians: A multicenter, randomized, parallel-group, delayed-start design study. Allergol Int 2018;67(2): 209–16.

82. Meglio P, Giampietro PG, Carello R, et al. Oral food desensitization in children with IgE-mediated hen's egg allergy: a new protocol with raw hen's egg. Pediatr Allergy Immunol 2013;24(1):75–83.

83. Martín-Muñoz MF, Belver MT, Alonso Lebrero E, et al. Egg oral immunotherapy in children (SEICAP I): Daily or weekly desensitization pattern. Pediatr Allergy Immunol 2019;30(1):81–92.

84. Martín-Muñoz MF, Alonso Lebrero E, Zapatero L, et al. Egg OIT in clinical practice (SEICAP II): Maintenance patterns and desensitization state after normalizing the diet. Pediatr Allergy Immunol 2019;30(2):214–24.

85. Buchanan AD, Green TD, Jones SM, et al. Egg oral immunotherapy in nonanaphylactic children with egg allergy. J Allergy Clin Immunol 2007;119(1):199–205.

86. Burks AW, Jones SM. Egg oral immunotherapy in non-anaphylactic children with egg allergy: follow-up. J Allergy Clin Immunol 2008;121(1):270–1.

87. Vickery BP, Pons L, Kulis M, et al. Individualized IgE-based dosing of egg oral immunotherapy and the development of tolerance. Ann Allergy Asthma Immunol 2010;105(6):444–50.

88. Yanagida N, Sato S, Asaumi T, et al. Safety and efficacy of low-dose oral immunotherapy for hen's egg allergy in children. Int Arch Allergy Immunol 2016; 171(3–4):265–8.

89. Maeta A, Matsushima M, Muraki N, et al. Low-dose oral immunotherapy using low-egg-allergen cookies for severe egg-allergic children reduces allergy severity and affects allergen-specific antibodies in serum. Int Arch Allergy Immunol 2018;175(1–2):70–6.

90. Bird JA, Clark A, Dougherty I, et al. Baked egg oral immunotherapy desensitizes baked egg allergic children to lightly cooked egg. J Allergy Clin Immunol Pract 2019;7(2):667–9, e4.

91. Staden U, Rolinck-Werninghaus C, Brewe F, et al. Specific oral tolerance induction in food allergy in children: efficacy and clinical patterns of reaction. Allergy 2007;62(11):1261–9.

92. Fuentes-Aparicio V, Alvarez-Perea A, Infante S, et al. Specific oral tolerance induction in paediatric patients with persistent egg allergy. Allergol Immunopathol (Madr) 2013;41(3):143–50.

93. Jeong HI, Lee B, Kim S, et al. Home-based up-dosing in build-up phase of oral immunotherapy of egg allergy is safe and feasible in real-world practice. Allergy Asthma Immunol Res 2021;13(5):791–8.

94. Akashi M, Yasudo H, Narita M, et al. Randomized controlled trial of oral immunotherapy for egg allergy in Japanese patients. Pediatr Int 2017;59(5):534–9.

95. Palosuo K, Karisola P, Savinko T, et al. A randomized, open-label trial of hen's egg oral immunotherapy: efficacy and humoral immune responses in 50 children. J Allergy Clin Immunol Pract 2021;9(5):1892–901.e1.

96. Romantsik O, Tosca MA, Zappettini S, et al. Oral and sublingual immunotherapy for egg allergy. Cochrane Database Syst Rev 2018;4:CD010638.

97. Kim EH, Jones SM, Burks AW, et al. A 5-year summary of real-life dietary egg consumption after completion of a 4-year egg powder oral immunotherapy (eOIT) protocol. J Allergy Clin Immunol 2020;145(4):1292–5.e1.

98. Clark A, Islam S, King Y, et al. A longitudinal study of resolution of allergy to well-cooked and uncooked egg. Clin Exp Allergy 2011;41(5):706–12.

99. Natsume O, Kabashima S, Nakazato J, et al. Two-step egg introduction for prevention of egg allergy in high-risk infants with eczema (PETIT): a randomised, double-blind, placebo-controlled trial. Lancet 2017;389(10066):276–86.

100. Bravin K, Luyt D. Home-based oral immunotherapy with a baked egg protocol. J Investig Allergol Clin Immunol 2016;26(1):61–3.

101. Gruzelle V, Juchet A, Martin-Blondel A, et al. Evaluation of baked egg oral immunotherapy in French children with hen's egg allergy. Pediatr Allergy Immunol 2021;32(5):1022–8.

102. Kim EH, Perry TT, Wood RA, et al. Induction of sustained unresponsiveness after egg oral immunotherapy compared to baked egg therapy in children with egg allergy. J Allergy Clin Immunol 2020;146(4):851–62, e10.

103. Rodríguez del Río P, Díaz-Perales A, Sanchez-García S, et al. Oral immunotherapy in children with IgE-mediated wheat allergy: outcome and molecular changes. J Investig Allergol Clin Immunol 2014;24(4):240–8.

104. Sato S, Utsunomiya T, Imai T, et al. Wheat oral immunotherapy for wheat-induced anaphylaxis. J Allergy Clin Immunol 2015;136(4):1131–3, e7.

105. Okada Y, Yanagida N, Sato S, et al. Better management of wheat allergy using a very low-dose food challenge: A retrospective study. Allergol Int 2016; 65(1):82–7.

106. Khayatzadeh A, Gharaghozlou M, Ebisawa M, et al. A safe and effective method for wheat oral immunotherapy. Iran J Allergy Asthma Immunol 2016;15(6): 525–35.

107. Rekabi M, Arshi S, Bemanian MH, et al. Evaluation of a new protocol for wheat desensitization in patients with wheat-induced anaphylaxis. Immunotherapy 2017;9(8):637–45.

108. Sharafian S, Amirzargar A, Gharagozlou M, et al. The efficacy of a new protocol of oral immunotherapy to wheat for desensitization and induction of tolerance. Iran J Allergy Asthma Immunol 2022;21(3):232–40.

109. Nowak-Węgrzyn A, Wood RA, Nadeau KC, et al. Multicenter, randomized, double-blind, placebo-controlled clinical trial of vital wheat gluten oral immunotherapy. J Allergy Clin Immunol 2019;143(2):651–61, e9.

110. Babaie D, Ebisawa M, Soheili H, et al. Oral wheat immunotherapy: long-term follow-up in children with wheat anaphylaxis. Int Arch Allergy Immunol 2022; 183(3):306–14.

111. Nagakura KI, Yanagida N, Miura Y, et al. Long-term follow-up of fixed low-dose oral immunotherapy for children with wheat-induced anaphylaxis. J Allergy Clin Immunol Pract 2022;10(4):1117–9.e2.

112. Nagakura KI, Yanagida N, Sato S, et al. Low-dose-oral immunotherapy for children with wheat-induced anaphylaxis. Pediatr Allergy Immunol 2020;31(4): 371–9.

113. Nachshon L, Goldberg MR, Levy MB, et al. Efficacy and safety of sesame oral immunotherapy-a real-world, single-center study. J Allergy Clin Immunol Pract 2019;7(8):2775–81.e2.

114. Elizur A, Appel MY, Nachshon L, et al. Cashew oral immunotherapy for desensitizing cashew-pistachio allergy (NUT CRACKER study). Allergy 2022;77(6): 1863–72.

115. Elizur A, Appel MY, Nachshon L, et al. Walnut oral immunotherapy for desensitisation of walnut and additional tree nut allergies (Nut CRACKER): a single-centre, prospective cohort study. Lancet Child Adolesc Health 2019;3(5): 312–21.

116. Moraly T, Pelletier de Chambure D, Verdun S, et al. Oral Immunotherapy for Hazelnut Allergy: A Single-Center Retrospective Study on 100 Patients. J Allergy Clin Immunol Pract 2020;8(2):704–9, e4.

117. Bégin P, Winterroth LC, Dominguez T, et al. Safety and feasibility of oral immunotherapy to multiple allergens for food allergy. Allergy Asthma Clin Immunol 2014;10(1):1.

118. Inuo C, Tanaka K, Suzuki S, et al. Oral immunotherapy using partially hydrolyzed formula for cow's milk protein allergy: a randomized, controlled trial. Int Arch Allergy Immunol 2018;177(3):259–68.

119. Lauener R, Eigenmann PA, Wassenberg J, et al. Oral immunotherapy with partially hydrolyzed wheat-based cereals: a pilot study. Clin Med Insights Pediatr 2017;11. 1179556517730018.

120. Tang ML, Ponsonby AL, Orsini F, et al. Administration of a probiotic with peanut oral immunotherapy: a randomized trial. J Allergy Clin Immunol 2015;135(3): 737–44, e8.

121. Srivastava KD, Siefert A, Fahmy TM, et al. Investigation of peanut oral immunotherapy with CpG/peanut nanoparticles in a murine model of peanut allergy. J Allergy Clin Immunol 2016;138(2):536–543 e4.

122. Chinthrajah S, Cao S, Liu C, et al. Phase 2a randomized, placebo-controlled study of anti-IL-33 in peanut allergy. JCI Insight 2019;4(22):e131347.

123. Fiocchi A, Vickery BP, Wood RA. The use of biologics in food allergy. Clin Exp Allergy 2021;51(8):1006–18.

124. Omalizumab as monotherapy and as adjunct therapy to multi-allergen OIT in food allergic participants (OUtMATCH). Available at: https://clinicaltrials.gov/ct2/show/NCT03881696. Accessed July 24, 2022.

125. Protection From food induced anaphylaxis by reducing the serum level of specific IgE (protana). Available at: https://clinicaltrials.gov/ct2/show/NCT03964051. Accessed July 24, 2022.

126. Omalizumab to accelerate a symptom-driven multi-food OIT (BOOM). Available at: https://clinicaltrials.gov/ct2/show/NCT04045301. Accessed July 24, 2022.

127. E-B-FAHF-2, Multi OIT and Xolair (Omalizumab) for Food Allergy. Available at: https://clinicaltrials.gov/ct2/show/NCT02879006. Accessed July 24, 2022.

128. Study in pediatric subjects with peanut allergy to evaluate efficacy and safety of dupilumab as adjunct to ar101 (peanut oral immunotherapy). Available at: https://clinicaltrials.gov/ct2/show/NCT03682770. Accessed July 24, 2022.

129. Study to evaluate dupilumab monotherapy in pediatric patients with peanut allergy. Available at: https://clinicaltrials.gov/ct2/show/NCT03793608. Accessed July 24, 2022.

130. Clinical study using biologics to improve multi OIT outcomes (COMBINE), Available at: https://clinicaltrials.gov/ct2/show/NCT03679676. Accessed July 24, 2022.

Eosinophilic Esophagitis
A Review for the Primary Care Practitioner

Alexandra Horwitz, MD[a], Samina Yunus, MD, MPH[b],*

KEYWORDS

- EoE review • Primary care practitioner • PCP • Esophageal • GERD and EoE

KEY POINTS

- Keep eosinophilic esophagitis in the differential diagnosis of a patient with upper gastrointestinal symptoms, especially in a patient with atopy.
- Recognize that the presentations may vary with age of the patient and the duration of disease.
- Refer appropriately for endoscopy/gastrointestinal evaluation if patient fails to respond to standard reflux therapy.
- A team effort with a nutritionist, gastroenterologist, and an allergist input will likely be needed.
- Monitor for compliance and complications of therapy.

EOSINOPHILIC ESOPHAGITIS
Introduction

Eosinophilic esophagitis (EoE) is a chronic antigen-mediated inflammatory disorder that is increasingly recognized as a cause of esophageal dysfunction in both adults and children.

Despite increased recognition of this condition, there can still be significant delays in time to diagnosis in both children and adults, which increases the risk of long-term morbidity, including fibrosis and strictures.[1]

Therefore, it is especially important for PCPs to be aware of the spectrum of clinical presentations, keep it in their differential diagnosis, and know how to screen for EoE symptoms in at-risk populations.

Epidemiology

Initially recognized as a distinct clinical entity in the mid-1990s,[2] it has since been increasingly seen as a major cause of esophageal dysfunction and as a source of significant health care burden both in terms of morbidity and cost.[3]

[a] Division of Allergy-Immunology, Penn State Health Children's Hospital, 90 Hope Drive, A480, Hershey, PA 17033, USA; [b] Case Western Reserve School of Medicine, Cleveland Clinic Department of Family Medicine, 551 East Washington Street, Chagrin Falls, OH 44023, USA
* Corresponding author.
E-mail address: yunuss@ccf.org

Prim Care Clin Office Pract 50 (2023) 283–294
https://doi.org/10.1016/j.pop.2022.11.004
0095-4543/23/© 2022 Elsevier Inc. All rights reserved.

The incidence of EoE is approximately 7.7/100,000 per year in adults and 6.6/100,000 per year in children.

EoE affects an estimated 34.4/100,000 people in Europe and North America. Since the mid-1990s there has been a significant increase in the overall prevalence of EoE for both age groups not fully explained by the increased recognition of the condition or change in diagnostic criteria.[4]

Prevalence rates in children increased from 19.1 (95% confidence interval [CI], 7.9–35.2) to 34.4 (95% CI, 22.3–49.2) patients per 100,000 inhabitants over 4 years, whereas for adults they grew from 32.5 (95% CI, 12.4–62.2) to 42.2 (95% CI, 31.1–55) patients per 100,000 inhabitants.[5]

Depending on the prevalence estimate, health care costs attributable to EoE range from $350 to $947 million/year.[3]

EoE can occur in any age group and has a 3:1 male to female predominance. The age at presentation is biphasic. The mean age at diagnosis in children is between 6 and 10 years, whereas in adults it occurs most commonly in the third and fourth decades.[6–8] There is an average delay in diagnosis of 4 years.

Most patients with EoE have an atopic history, and heritability has been established, with a recent multicenter analysis showing that 6.5% of patients had a parent or a sibling with EoE.[5]

In adult EoE patients, the prevalence of any atopic condition is 20% to 80%.[9] Children with EoE have a prevalence of 30% to 50% and 50% to 75% for asthma and allergic rhinitis. Furthermore, children with EoE are more likely to have environmental allergies and immunoglobulin E (IgE)-mediated food allergy (eg, urticaria, anaphylaxis). Moreover, a family history of an atopic disorder is found in more than 50% of patients with EoE.[10,11]

EoE also develops in association with some inherited connective tissue disorders that exhibit hypermobility, but this is rare.[12]

A family history of EoE increases an individual's risk for the condition.[13] Interestingly, the risk varies by the particular relationship with a higher risk if the father or brother is affected. A father affected gives a 2.4% individual risk (recurrence risk ratio: 43), and a brother affected gives a 3.5% individual risk (recurrence risk ratio: 64).[14]

DISCUSSION
Clinical Presentation

The clinical presentation of the individual patient to the PCP may be varied depending on the age of the patient, chronicity of disease, and prior treatments (**Table 1**). Solid food dysphagia and food impaction are more common in adults and adolescents and nausea, vomiting, heart burn, and abdominal pain in younger children. It is also a differential in exercise-induced chest pain in adults.[15] Failure to thrive and feeding refusal is seen in infants and toddlers. Food impaction has a high correlation with EoE, with studies demonstrating up to 36% of individuals presenting with food impaction having EoE.[16]

When assessing for dysphagia it is important to recognize that many patients may have subconsciously developed compensatory eating behaviors over years to minimize symptoms. So close questioning on eating habits is important to elicit. It is important to ask whether the patient has been eating slowly, chewing excessively, drinking copious amounts of fluids, repeating swallows, avoiding certain foods, and crushing or avoiding pills.

Making the diagnosis further challenging is the overlap of gastrointestinal reflux disease (GERD) and EoE as well as subset of patients with EoE who respond to PPIs. Therefore, a high index of suspicion must be maintained by the PCP in patients who

Table 1
Most common presenting symptoms of eosinophilic esophagitis by age

Age	Infants/Younger Children	Older Children/ Adolescents	Adults
Symptoms	Feeding refusal	Preference for soft/	Dysphagia
	Delayed feeding skills	liquid diet	Chest/upper abdominal
	Textural preferences	Heartburn	pain
	Vomiting chronic	Abdominal pain	Heartburn
	nausea/abdominal	Vomiting	
	pain	Dysphagia/choking/	
	Regurgitation	food sticking	
	Irritability	Fear/anxiety with meal	
		Food impaction	

are refractory to standard therapy for GERD and have commonly associated conditions or present with food impaction.

Pathophysiology

Major players in the pathology of eosinophilic esophagitis are activated eosinophils, mast cells, and Th2 cytokines. This disease does not seem to be IgE mediated (**Fig. 1**).[17]

An impaired esophageal epithelial barrier initiates a cascade of self-propagating events. Increased permeability of the esophageal lining is theorized due to altered functioning of desmoglein-1, calpain 14, and eotaxin. The increased presence of thymic stromal lymphopoietin acts on the antigen-presenting cells and induces CD4 cells to differentiate into mainly Th2 (T helper cells) and to a lesser extent Th1 cells.

Activated eosinophils in the epithelium release T-cell–activating cytokines, which induce Th2 cell differentiation and also degranulate and release preformed granule proteins. The preformed granules include eosinophil cationic protein, major basic protein, eosinophil peroxidase, and eosinophil-derived neurotoxin, which cause inflammation and edema. In addition, along with mast cells, eosinophils release TGF-β1, which stimulates epithelial cells to undergo mesenchymal changes causing subepithelial fibrosis. Eosinophils also release vascular cell adhesion molecule, which increases angiogenesis.[18]

Antigen-presenting cells and T-cell–activating cytokines induce the differentiation of CD4 cells both locally and systemically. Activated Th2 cells release interleukin-4 (IL-4), IL-5, and IL-13. IL-4 recruits mast cells that release histamine, cytokines, serine proteases (tryptase, chymase), and proteoglycans causing local inflammation. Mast cells also release TGF-β1, which induces epithelial fibrosis. IL-4 also induces release of periostin, a profibrotic agent. IL-5 is a key cytokine involved in proliferation and survival of eosinophils. IL-13 induces the secretion of eotaxin in the esophageal epithelium, which increases the recruitment, retention, and activation of eosinophils to the esophagus. It also induces the secretion of proteolytic enzymes calpain 14, desmoglein, and filaggrin affecting epithelial integrity.[19]

Evaluation and Diagnosis

Patients who present with any of the aforementioned symptoms should be further queried about all the potential symptoms of EoE. It is also helpful to ask about risk factors for EoE, such as a personal history of other atopic conditions, even if resolved,

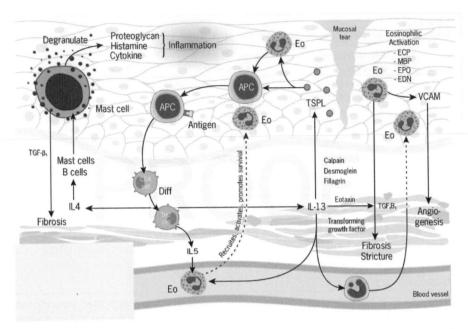

Fig. 1. Pathophysiology of eosinophilic esophagitis. APC, antigen presenting cell; ECP, eosin-ophilic cationic protein; EDN, eosinophil derived neurotoxin; Eo, eosinophil; E-PO, eosino-phil peroxidase; MBP, major basic protein; TSLP, thymic stromal lymphopoeitin; VCAM, vascular cell adhesion molecule. (Reprinted with permission, Cleveland Clinic Foundation ©2022. All Rights Reserved.)

and any family history of EoE, severe GERD, food impactions/dysphagia, or need for esophageal dilatations.

Patients who may present for routine preventative care and have conditions asso-ciated with an increased risk of EoE should be screened with a targeted review of systems for evidence of dysphagia and the other gastrointestinal manifestations of EoE.

All patients suspected of having EoE should be referred to gastroenterology for an esophagogastroduodenoscopy (EGD) to establish the diagnosis. Although not diag-nostic, certain gross endoscopic findings are frequently seen in patients with EoE. These include Exudates, Rings, Edema, Furrows, Strictures, and trachealization. The first 4 findings are used to generate an eosinophilic esophagitis endoscopic refer-ence score (**Table 2**), which is a classification system used routinely in clinical practice to assess severity of disease. However, biopsy is necessary to establish the diagnosis and assess response to treatment.[20–22] Maximum sensitivity is achieved by obtaining multiple biopsies from proximal and/or mid- and distal esophagus.

Original diagnostic criteria required that eosinophils be present despite the patient being on a high-dose proton pump inhibitor (PPI) for 8 weeks. However, this criterion was removed in the updated guidelines in 2018 due to evidence that EoE and GERD can co-exist and perhaps potentiate each other. Some patients with EoE and no ev-idence of GERD respond to PPIs (formerly known as PPI-responsive esophageal eosinophilia, now classified as a subset of EoE), and PPIs have a nonacid–mediated mechanism of action that contributes to their effectiveness in EoE.

Table 2
Eosinophilic esophagitis endoscopic reference scores

Major Features			Minor Features		
Fixed rings	Grade 0	None	Crepe-paper esophagus (mucosal fragility or laceration passage of endoscope)	Grade 0	Absent
	Grade 1	Mild (subtle circumferential ridges)		Grade 1	Present
	Grade 2	Moderate (distinct rings, permits passage of endoscope)			
	Grade 3	Severe (distinct rings, do not permit passage, of endoscope)			
Exudates	Grade 0	None			
	Grade 1	Mild (<10% of the esophageal surface area)			
	Grade 2	Severe (>10% of the esophageal surface area)			
Edema	Grade 0	Absent (distinct vascularity present)			
	Grade 1	Loss of clarity or absence of vascular markings			
Furrows	Grade 0	Absent			
	Grade 1	Present			
Stricture	Grade 0	Absent			
	Grade 1	Present			

From Hirano I, Moy N, Heckman MG, Thomas CS, Gonsalves N, Achem SR. Endoscopic assessment of the oesophageal features of eosinophilic oesophagitis: validation of a novel classification and grading system. Gut. 2013;62(4):489-495.

Criteria for Diagnosis

Criteria for diagnosis are based on the AGREE[23] group consensus statement from 2018 and has 3 components:

1. Clinical symptoms of esophageal dysfunction;
2. An esophageal eosinophil count of more than or equal to 15 eosinophils/high-power field, and
3. Exclusion of other possible causes of esophageal eosinophilia.

Differential Diagnosis

It is important to be aware of other causes of esophageal eosinophilia as well as the possibility of a concurrent diagnosis. The differential is quite broad; however, GERD is the most common condition that can not only mimic but also coexist with EoE. Other conditions in the differential diagnosis include achalasia, eosinophilic gastrointestinal disease, hyper eosinophilic syndrome, Crohn disease, celiac disease, vasculitis, connective tissue disorders, and infections.

Management

The goal of therapy is both symptomatic and histologic resolution of symptoms and reduction in the long-term sequelae of untreated EoE.

Table 3
AAAAI/ACAAI joint task force on allergy/immunology practice parameters and AGA release guideline on the management of eosinophilic esophagitis

Recommendation	Strength of Recommendation	Quality of Evidence
In patients with EoE, the AGA/JTF recommends topical glucocorticosteroids over no treatment	Strong	Moderate
In patients with EoE, the AGA/JTF suggests topical glucocorticosteroids rather than oral glucocorticosteroids	Conditional	Moderate
In patients with EoE, the AGA/JTF suggests using elemental diet over no treatment	Conditional	Moderate
In patients with EoE, the AGA/JTF suggests using an empirical, 6-food elimination diet over no treatment	Conditional	Low
Testing-based elimination diet over no treatment	Conditional	Very low
In patients with EoE in remission after short-term topical glucocorticosteroids, the AGA/JTF suggests continuation of topical glucocorticosteroids over discontinuation	Conditional	Very low
In adult patients with dysphagia from a very low-quality endoscopic dilation over no dilation	Conditional	Very low
In patients with EoE, the AGA/JTF recommends using anti-IL-5 therapy for EoE only in the context of a clinical trial	No recommendation	Knowledge gap
In patients with EoE, the AGA/JTF recommends using anti-IL-13 or anti-IL-4 receptor therapy for EoE only in the context of a clinical trial[a]	No recommendation	Knowledge gap
In patients with EoE, the AGA/JTF suggests against the use of anti-IgE therapy for EoE	Conditional	Very low
In patients with EoE the AGA/JTF suggests using montelukast, cromolyn sodium, immunomodulators, and anti-TNF for EoE only in the context of a clinical trial	No recommendation	Knowledge gap

Abbreviation: TNF, tumor necrosis factor.
[a] Dupixent is an anti-IL-4, IL-13 agent FDA approved on May 20, 2022.

As with most chronic disease management, a patient-centered approach with treatment streamlined to make it as nondisruptive to the patients as possible is preferred. Which treatment strategy is chosen is based on shared decision-making between the practitioners and family. In addition, a multidisciplinary approach with a team composed of an allergist, a gastroenterologist, a dietitian, and the primary care practitioner is preferred.

New guidelines were released in 2020 from the American Gastroenterological Association (AGA) and the Joint Task Force for Allergy-Immunology Practice Parameters, which provided recommendations for the management of EoE in pediatric and adult patients (**Table 3**). The only strong recommendation was the recommendation for the use of topical steroids over no treatment. The rest of the recommendations were conditional and included use of PPIs over no treatment, use of topical rather than systemic steroids, and the use of elemental, empirical elimination diets or allergy testing–based elimination diet over no treatment. Importantly, continuing treatment after remission was also a conditional recommendation.[24]

Use of anti-IL-3, IL-4, or IL-5, montelukast, and antitumor necrosis factor therapy was only recommended in the context of clinical trials, and anti-IgE therapy was not recommended.[24] *Of note, as of May 2022, dupilumab (anti-IL-4/IL-13) was granted Food and Drug Administration (FDA) approval for the treatment of EoE in those 12 years and older.*

The 3 main modalities currently in use for EoE are diet, medications, and endoscopic dilatation (**Table 4**).

Dietary Modalities

- Elemental diets consisting of exclusively amino acid–based formula are highly effective—93.6% resolution compared with placebo (13.3%) in 6 observational studies.[5] However, they are difficult to sustain and poorly palatable. A disruption of children's developmental feeding progress and need for gastrostomy tubes are possible downsides.[5,25]
- Empirical elimination diets consist of removing food groups that are commonly implicated in EoE (**Table 5**). The traditional 6-food elimination diet includes elimination of milk, wheat, soy, egg, nuts, and fish/seafood from diet. This induces remission in approximately 67% of patents compared with 13% with placebo noted in 9 observational studies. It requires repeated endoscopy to assess for response, as each food group is then reintroduced. Elimination diets of 2 and 4 food are less effective[5,26]; however, a recent study looked at a step-up approach to therapy in which participants began with a 2-food elimination diet (milk, gluten) and if no response after 6 weeks, went to a 4-food elimination. Nonresponders at 6 weeks then went to the 6-food elimination. The results showed remission rates of 43% with 2-food elimination, 60% with 4-food elimination, and 79% with 6-food elimination, with greater than 90% of the 2- and 4-food group responders having 1 to 2 food triggers. Endoscopic procedures and diagnostic times were reduced by 20% with this step-up strategy.[27]
- Allergy testing–based elimination diets consist of eliminating foods that are positive on skin and/or atopy patch testing. Because EoE is not IgE mediated and atopy patch testing for foods is not standardized, this is less effective than the previous 2 dietary approaches. However, 50.8% of patients respond to this approach compared with 13.3% to placebo. This approach has largely fallen out of favor.

Medications

Before May 2022 there were no medications approved by FDA for EoE. In May 2022 dupilumab, a monoclonal antibody against IL-4 and IL-13, became the first FDA-approved medication for the treatment of EoE in patients older than 12 years and 40 kg (88 lbs) in weight. Topical steroids and PPIs are most commonly used for first-line management.

Topical Steroids

Topical steroids include either fluticasone via inhaler swallowed 88 to 440 μg twice daily in children and 440 to 880 ug twice daily in adults, or oral viscous budesonide (budesonide nebulizer solution mixed in vehicle such as honey, applesauce, maple syrup, or sucralose to make slurry), 0.5 to 1 mg twice daily in children and 1 to 2 mg in adults. They have shown to induce remission in 65% of patients versus 13.3% with placebo.

It is important to be aware of the risk of esophageal candidiasis with this therapy and treat the patient appropriately should they develop odynophagia.

Table 4
Current treatment options for eosinophilic esophagitis

	Treatment	Mode of Action	Dose	Formulation	Efficacy vs Placebo	Side Effects	Clinical Considerations
Diet[a]	Elemental	Avoids allergen	Individualized	Amino acid–based formula	93.60%	Unpalatable	Needs support to ensure adherence; cost; IgE-mediated food sensitivity on reintroduction
	6-food Elimination diet	Avoids allergen	—	Eliminate milk, wheat, soy, egg, nuts, fish/seafood	67.90%	—	Needs support to ensure adherence; dairy and wheat are the most common culprits.
	Allergy testing–based elimination diet	Avoids allergen	—	Eliminate allergens in diet	50.80%	—	Needs patient motivation, less effective than 6-food elimination
Drugs	Proton pump inhibitors	Anti-inflammatory omeprazole maintains mucosal integrity	20 mg BID	Capsule	41.70%	Diarrhea including cliff	Easily available, low-cost, well-tolerated needs higher doses than in treatment of GERD
Tropical corticosteroids	Fluticasone	Anti-inflammatory	440–880 UG BID	Inhaler-swallow	64.90%	Oral and esophageal candidiasis	Adrenal suppression off-label use.
	Budesonide Dupilumab	— Biological anti-IL-4 and IL-13	1–2 mg BID 300 mg weekly	Slurry Subcutaneous injection	— 60.00%	— Respiratory infection arthralgia	12 y and clear weighing at least 40 kg. Avoid live vaccines; pregnancy registry

a See text for additional diets.

Table 5	
Common food triggers in eosinophilic esophagitis	
Children	**Adults**
• Milk	• Wheat
• Wheat	• Milk
• Egg	• Soy
• Soy	• Egg
• Corn ("other grains")	• Corn ("other grains")
• Beef ("meats")	• Beef ("meats")

Adrenal suppression (1.4%) with a higher dose of 2 mg bid of budesonide has been reported in a cohort of 318 patients followed-up for 8 weeks.[5]

Proton Pump Inhibitors

PPIs are traditionally needed in higher doses than in the management of GERD and result in remission in approximately 41% of patient's versus 13.3% with placebo.[5] PPIs both maintain mucosal integrity by reducing acidity and are also proposed to have antiinflammatory effect by reducing release of eotaxin-3 in response to IL-13[28] (**Fig. 2**).

Endoscopy with Dilatation

Endoscopy with dilatation is needed in more advanced stenotic disease. Dilatation provides immediate and long-term relief but does not address the underlying process. There is risk of esophageal perforation but much less than initially thought. The optimal role of dilatation is controversial.

Monitoring Therapy

Current criteria for monitoring treatment response requires an endoscopy after initiation of treatment and after changes in treatment; however, less invasive procedures to assess response and esophageal function show promise.[5]

Assessment of response has been demonstrated with use of an esophageal capsule with mesh attached to a string for esophageal scrapings, an esophageal string, or transnasal endoscopy as alternatives to traditional endoscopy. Esophageal function can be assessed using a gene sequence or functional luminal imaging probe a US FDA–approved measuring tool to measure pressure and distensibility of the esophagus and risk of stenosis.[5] There are no guidelines for routine EGD surveillance after remission has been achieved.

Duration of Therapy

Current guidelines favor ongoing treatment, as there is disease recurrence when treatment is discontinued. Therefore, close monitoring of patients by either the PCP, allergist, or gastroenterologist for adherence to treatment, recurrence of symptoms, and possible side effects and complications of therapy is needed.

SUMMARY

With the increase in prevalence of EoE in the general population, this is a condition primary care practitioners will increasingly encounter in their practice. Increased awareness of the condition, maintaining a high index of suspicion, appropriate referral for endoscopy, and partnering with the patient and with specialists in gastroenterology and allergy immunology are essential to provide the best clinical outcome.

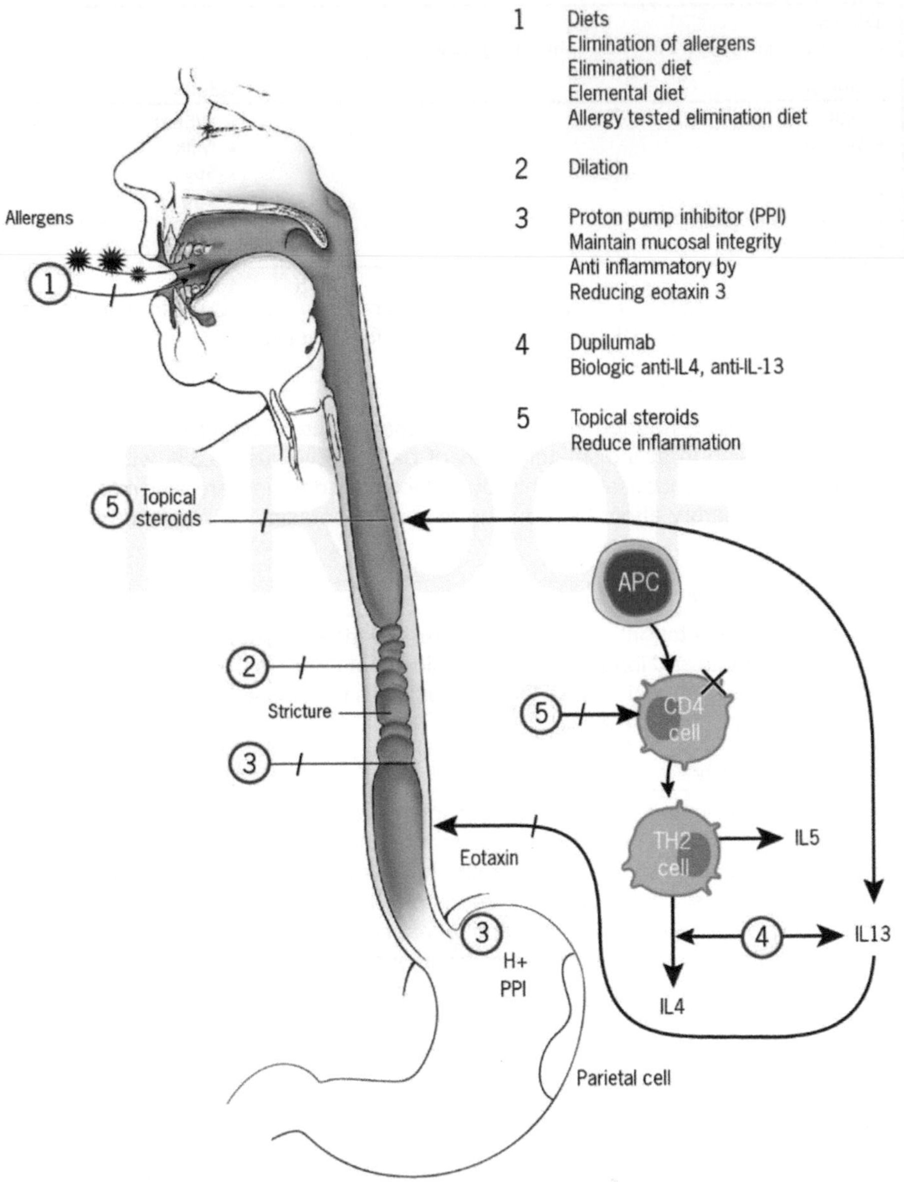

Fig. 2. Mechanism of action of medications eosinophilic esophagitis. (Reprinted with permission, Cleveland Clinic Foundation ©2022. All Rights Reserved.)

CLINICS CARE POINTS

- Keep EoE in mind when patients present with symptoms such as dysphagia, food impaction, unexplained vomiting, abdominal pain, food refusal, or failure to thrive, especially if they have other atopic conditions.
- Keep EoE in mind in patients with GERD that is refractory to standard treatment.

- Screen periodically for EoE in patients with atopic conditions.
- Gastroenterology referral is needed for diagnosis by EGD with biopsies; allergists can suspect and help manage but cannot diagnose EoE.
- The most common trigger foods are milk, wheat, egg, soy, grains, and meats. There are numerous dietary elimination options, but with all, adherence is challenging and nutritional support is critical.
- PPIs are now considered an effective treatment option for EoE and are safe.
- Dupilumab is an FDA-approved medication for patients aged 12 years and older and who weigh at least 40 kg (88 lbs).

DISCLOSURE

The authors have nothing to disclose.

REFERENCES

1. Dellon E, Aderoju A, Woosley J, et al. Variability in Diagnostic Criteria for Eosinophilic Esophagitis: A Systematic Review. Am J Gastroenterol 2007;102(10): 2300–13. https://doi.org/10.1111/j.1572-0241.2007.01396.
2. Schoepfer A, Safroneeva E, Bussmann C, et al. Delay in Diagnosis of Eosinophilic Esophagitis Increases Risk for Stricture Formation in a Time-Dependent Manner. Gastroenterology 2013;145(6):1230–6.e2. https://doi.org/10.1053/j.gastro.2013. 08.015.
3. Jensen E, Kappelman M, Martin C, et al. Health-Care Utilization, Costs, and the Burden of Disease Related to Eosinophilic Esophagitis in the United States. Am J Gastroenterol 2015;110(5):626–32. https://doi.org/10.1038/ajg.2014.316.
4. Navarro P, Arias Á, Arias-González L, et al. Systematic review with meta-analysis: the growing incidence and prevalence of eosinophilic oesophagitis in children and adults in population-based studies. Aliment Pharmacol Ther 2019;49(9): 1116–25. https://doi.org/10.1111/apt.15231.
5. Muir A, Falk G. Eosinophilic Esophagitis. JAMA 2021;326(13):1310. https://doi. org/10.1001/jama.2021.14920.
6. Bystrom J, O'Shea N. Eosinophilic oesophagitis: clinical presentation and pathogenesis. Postgrad Med J 2014;90(1063):282–9. https://doi.org/10.1136/ postgradmedj-2012-131403.
7. Markowitz J, Clayton S. Eosinophilic Esophagitis in Children and Adults. Gastrointest Endosc Clin N Am 2018;28(1):59–75. https://doi.org/10.1016/j.giec.2017.07.004.
8. Lucendo A, Molina-Infante J, Arias Á, et al. Guidelines on eosinophilic esophagitis: evidence-based statements and recommendations for diagnosis and management in children and adults. United Eur Gastroenterol J 2017;5(3):335–58. https://doi.org/10.1177/2050640616689525.
9. Dellon E, Liacouras C. Advances in Clinical Management of Eosinophilic Esophagitis. Gastroenterology 2014;147(6):1238–54. https://doi.org/10.1053/j.gastro. 2014.07.055.
10. Simon D, Marti H, Heer P, et al. Eosinophilic esophagitis is frequently associated with IgE-mediated allergic airway diseases. J Allergy Clin Immunol 2005;115(5): 1090–2. https://doi.org/10.1016/j.jaci.2005.01.017.
11. Assa'ad A. Eosinophilic Esophagitis: Association with Allergic Disorders. Gastrointest Endosc Clin N Am 2008;18(1):119–32. https://doi.org/10.1016/j.giec.2007. 09.001.

12. Abonia J, Wen T, Stucke E, et al. High prevalence of eosinophilic esophagitis in patients with inherited connective tissue disorders. J Allergy Clin Immunol 2013; 132(2):378–86. https://doi.org/10.1016/j.jaci.2013.02.030.

13. Noel R, Putnam P, Rothenberg M. Eosinophilic Esophagitis. N Engl J Med 2004; 351(9):940–1. https://doi.org/10.1056/nejm200408263510924.

14. Reed C, Dellon E. Eosinophilic Esophagitis. Med Clin North Am 2019;103(1): 29–42. https://doi.org/10.1016/j.mcna.2018.08.009.

15. Visaggi P, Savarino E, Sciume G, et al. Eosinophilic esophagitis: clinical, endoscopic, histologic and therapeutic differences and similarities between children and adults. Therap Adv Gastroenterol 2021;14. https://doi.org/10.1177/1756284820980860. 175628482098086.

16. Lenz C, Leggett C, Katzka D, et al. Food impaction: etiology over 35 years and association with eosinophilic esophagitis. Dis Esophagus 2018;32(4). https://doi.org/10.1093/dote/doy093.

17. Clayton F, Fang J, Gleich G, et al. Eosinophilic esophagitis in adults is associated with IgG4 and Not Mediated by IgE. Gastroenterology 2014;147(3):602–9. https://doi.org/10.1053/j.gastro.2014.05.036.

18. Raheem M, Leach S, Day A, et al. The Pathophysiology of Eosinophilic Esophagitis. Front Pediatr 2014;2. https://doi.org/10.3389/fped.2014.00041.

19. Gómez-Aldana A, Jaramillo-Santos M, Delgado A, et al. Eosinophilic esophagitis: Current concepts in diagnosis and treatment. World J Gastroenterol 2019;25(32): 4598–613. https://doi.org/10.3748/wjg.v25.i32.4598.

20. Hirano I, Aceves S. Clinical Implications and Pathogenesis of Esophageal Remodeling in Eosinophilic Esophagitis. Gastroenterol Clin North Am 2014;43(2): 297–316. https://doi.org/10.1016/j.gtc.2014.02.015.

21. Alexander J. Endoscopic and Radiologic Findings in Eosinophilic Esophagitis. Gastrointest Endosc Clin N Am 2018;28(1):47–57. https://doi.org/10.1016/j.giec.2017.07.003.

22. Hirano I, Moy N, Heckman M, et al. Endoscopic assessment of the oesophageal features of eosinophilic oesophagitis: validation of a novel classification and grading system. Gut 2012;62(4):489–95. https://doi.org/10.1136/gutjnl-2011-301817.

23. Dellon E, Liacouras C, Molina-Infante J, et al. Updated International Consensus Diagnostic Criteria for Eosinophilic Esophagitis: Proceedings of the AGREE Conference. Gastroenterology 2018;155(4):1022–33.e10. https://doi.org/10.1053/j.gastro.2018.07.009.

24. Hirano I, Chan E, Rank M, et al. AGA Institute and the Joint Task Force on Allergy-Immunology Practice Parameters Clinical Guidelines for the Management of Eosinophilic Esophagitis. Gastroenterology 2020;158(6):1776–86. https://doi.org/10.1053/j.gastro.2020.02.038.

25. Warners M, Vlieg-Boerstra B, Verheij J, et al. Elemental diet decreases inflammation and improves symptoms in adult eosinophilic oesophagitis patients. Aliment Pharmacol Ther 2017;45(6):777–87. https://doi.org/10.1111/apt.13953.

26. Gonsalves N, Yang G, Doerfler B, et al. Elimination Diet Effectively Treats Eosinophilic Esophagitis in Adults; Food Reintroduction Identifies Causative Factors. Gastroenterology 2012;142(7). https://doi.org/10.1053/j.gastro.2012.03.001. 1451-9.e1.

27. Molina-Infante J, Gonzalez-Cordero P, Casabona-Frances S, et al. Step-Up Empiric Elimination Diet for Pediatric and Adult Eosinophilic Esophagitis: The 2-4-6 Study. Gastroenterology 2017;152(5):S207. https://doi.org/10.1016/s0016-5085(17)30998-8.

28. Eluri S, Dellon E. Proton pump inhibitor-responsive oesophageal eosinophilia and eosinophilic oesophagitis. Curr Opin Gastroenterol 2015;31(4):309–15. https://doi.org/10.1097/mog.0000000000000185.

Hereditary Angioedema
A Disease Often Misdiagnosed and Mistreated

Arindam Sarkar, MD[a],*, Crystal Nwagwu, MD[a],
Timothy Craig, DO[b]

KEYWORDS

- Hereditary angioedema • Bradykinin • C1 inhibitor

KEY POINTS

- Hereditary angioedema (HAE) is often overlooked or misdiagnosed. It is associated with significant morbidity and potential mortality.
- HAE presents with recurrent attacks of subcutaneous and submucosal swelling without urticaria.
- Unlike the more common histamine-mediated causes of angioedema, HAE is bradykinin-mediated and refractory to antihistamines, epinephrine, and corticosteroids.
- Appropriate therapy requires drugs specific to the excess release of bradykinin.

BACKGROUND

Hereditary angioedema (HAE) is a rare, inherited condition characterized by recurrent episodes of nonpruritic, nonpitting swelling typically involving the skin, intestinal wall, genitalia, and upper airway. Generally, angioedema is a clinical syndrome marked by a rapid increase in vascular permeability of submucosal and subcutaneous (SC) tissues. Although angioedema is most commonly mediated by histamine, HAE specifically depends on the release of bradykinin. There are several clinical and pathophysiological features that differentiate HAE from mast-cell mediated swelling typical of allergic reactions.

Lack of physician awareness of HAE and overlapping clinical features of angioedema with histamine-mediated or medication-induced angioedema can make a timely diagnosis challenging. In a 2010 study, 313 patients with HAE reported visiting an average of 4.4 physicians over an average of 8.3 years before receiving an accurate HAE diagnosis.[1] These diagnostic delays have been associated with psychosocial distress, unnecessary surgeries, and even death. In a cohort of 728 patients with a

---

[a] Department of Family and Community Medicine, Baylor College of Medicine, 1100 West 34th Street, Houston, TX 77007, USA; [b] Pediatrics and Biomedical Sciences, Penn State University, 500 University Drive, Hershey, PA 17033, USA
* Corresponding author.
E-mail address: arindams@bcm.edu
Twitter: @arindammd (A.S.)

Prim Care Clin Office Pract 50 (2023) 295–303
https://doi.org/10.1016/j.pop.2022.11.005
0095-4543/23/© 2022 Elsevier Inc. All rights reserved.

family history of HAE, 214 premature deaths were described. One-third of the deaths were from laryngeal edema and subsequent asphyxiation (N = 70) and 63 of those subjects died before HAE was diagnosed.[2]

Although rare, HAE is a debilitating and potentially life-threatening disease. Medications such as epinephrine, antihistamines, or glucocorticoid therapies do not provide relief and often delay care. Through broader physician awareness, earlier diagnosis and initiation of prophylaxis therapy can significantly reduce the morbidity and mortality of HAE. The following discussion reviews the diagnostic and therapeutic considerations in the approach to a patient with HAE.

DISCUSSION
Pathophysiology

HAE is an autosomal dominant disorder without predominance in any ethnicity or gender.[3] With an estimated frequency of 1 per 50,000 Americans, HAE is considered rare.[4] HAE presents with attacks of SC and submucosal swelling in the respiratory and gastrointestinal tracts. These episodes result from either low levels or improper function of a protein called C1 esterase inhibitor (often abbreviated to C1-inhibitor or C1-INH).

There are 3 types of HAE. In type I, which represents 80% to 85% of cases, a deficiency of circulating C1-INH manifests in attacks. In type II, which represents 15% of cases, reduced functional levels of C1-INH cause similar symptoms.[5] HAE with normal C1-INH (previously referred to as type III HAE) is extremely rare. The mechanism for these cases is not well understood and will not be included in this discussion.

The C1-INH protein acts within many pathways but is most clinically relevant to HAE within the contact activation system and the complement cascade. The contact activation system, also called the contact system or the kinin-kallikrein system, represents a growing area of research during the last 4 decades. The contact system has been implicated in blood pressure control, coagulation, and pain.[6] In the context of HAE, C1-INH normally inhibits kallikrein and activation of factor XII (sometimes called Hageman factor). A lack of C1-INH results in autoactivation of factor XII and activation of prekallikrein to kallikrein. Active kallikrein causes breakdown of high molecular weight kininogen, which subsequently produces a vasoactive peptide called bradykinin. Bradykinin acts on BR2 receptors leading to increased vascular permeability and angioedema.[7] In sum, when C1-INH is deficient or dysfunctional, uncontrolled bradykinin action causes HAE (**Fig. 1**).

In the classical complement pathway, C1-INH blocks activation of C1. C1 goes on to form the C1 complex, which cleaves C4. The result of both C1-INH deficiency (type I HAE) and dysfunction (type II HAE) is a low C4 level. Although C4 is not directly related to the clinical manifestations of HAE, the detection of low C4 levels is a useful and sensitive test (approximately 90%) for HAE.

Briefly, there is an additional role of C1-INH in the fibrinolytic system. The clinical relevance of that pathway to HAE is that D-dimer may be elevated during acute attacks (**Fig. 2**).

Clinical Manifestations

It is hypothesized that the degree of C1-INH deficiency or dysfunctionality plays a role in age of symptom onset, frequency of episodes, and severity of attacks. Approximately one-third of patients with type I or II HAE experience symptoms by age 5. Most cases present before 20 years of age, whereas an estimated 4% of patients will experience their first attack after age 40.[8] Some patients report many attacks

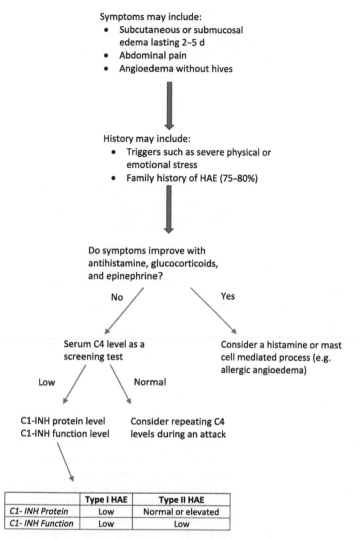

Symptoms may include:
- Subcutaneous or submucosal edema lasting 2–5 d
- Abdominal pain
- Angioedema without hives

History may include:
- Triggers such as severe physical or emotional stress
- Family history of HAE (75–80%)

Do symptoms improve with antihistamine, glucocorticoids, and epinephrine?

No / Yes

Serum C4 level as a screening test

Consider a histamine or mast cell mediated process (e.g. allergic angioedema)

Low / Normal

C1-INH protein level
C1-INH function level

Consider repeating C4 levels during an attack

	Type I HAE	Type II HAE
C1- INH Protein	Low	Normal or elevated
C1- INH Function	Low	Low

Fig. 1. An overview of the diagnostic approach to a patient with symptoms suggestive of hereditary angioedema. Notes: Low C4 should be repeated 1 to 3 month apart to confirm diagnosis.

each month, and some patients will go months without an attack. Uncommonly, an individual with HAE may never experience an attack.[3] An individual attack typically lasts 2 to 5 days. Attacks can be triggered by an emotionally or physically stressful circumstance, such as a wedding, athletic event or medical procedure. Older adults with symptoms similar to HAE may have a related condition called acquired angioedema with low C1-INH (AAE). AAE is also characterized by C1-INH deficiency, usually from an autoantibody.

Most patients experience swelling in specific parts of the body, although swelling can occur anywhere. Typically, HAE attacks manifest with upper airway, gastrointestinal, or cutaneous symptoms.[4] Laryngeal attacks are the least common but most dangerous type of attack due to airway obstruction with potential of asphyxiation. In

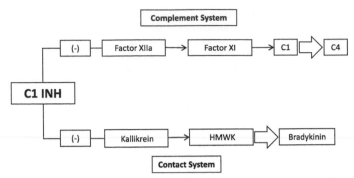

Fig. 2. A simplified summary of the role C1-INH in the contact system (kinin-kallikrein pathway) and the complement system as related to HAE. Dysfunctional or deficient C1-INH results in loss of regulation of factor XIIa and kallikrein. This leads to excess production of bradykinin. Bradykinin is the key molecule that mediates clinical manifestations of HAE.

a series of 138 patients with HAE, approximately half experienced an upper airway attack during their lifetime. This varied from mild tongue swelling to the formidable laryngeal edema. Upper airway edema has been reported to account for up to 33% of mortality in persons with HAE.[9]

Gastrointestinal attacks similarly range from mild to severe in intensity. Symptoms usually resolve without serious complications unless a patient undergoes unnecessary interventions because the disorder is not recognized as HAE. Cutaneous attacks are not associated with high risk of complications or death, although they may cause substantial lifestyle and occupational disruptions from recurrent bouts causing cosmetic concerns and disability (eg, hand swelling and unable to drive, foot swelling and inability to walk, facial disfigurement; **Table 1**).

Evaluation/Diagnosis

A diagnosis of HAE should be suspected in patients with recurrent attacks of angioedema to the face or airway—with or without abdominal pain. Importantly, C1-INH deficiency does not present with urticaria, also known as hives, wheals, or itching. In suspected cases, laboratory investigation should begin with a serum C4 level and then a C1 level and function. The C4 test has been documented to have a 100% sensitivity and a very high negative predictive value during an attack. Between attacks, the sensitivity has been described as 85% to 95%.[10] If C4 levels are low, the next steps are to check C1-INH levels and C1-INH protein functionality.

Although a complement C4 level is a very good screening test, most experts suggest obtaining C4 levels, C1-INH protein, and C1-INH function in all cases suggestive of HAE to avoid diagnostic ambiguity. A normal result on any one test does not rule out HAE as special sample handling requirements can affect results.[11]

Genetic testing is available to confirm the diagnosis of HAE. However, as biochemical tests are very effective in making the diagnosis for type 1 and 2 HAE, genetic testing is rarely necessary. The exceptions are if prenatal diagnosis is desired or if biochemical testing is equivocal during the first year of life. Most type I and II HAE cases are caused by mutations in the C1-inhibitor gene, *SERPING1*.[10] Because there are innumerable mutations in *SERPING1* gene, many that have not been identified, genetic testing is imperfect. In addition, other genes can result in an HAE with normal C1-inhibitor diagnosis, and thus universal genetic testing would have low clinical value. Presently, genetic testing is not recommended in patients with classic symptoms and a strong family history.[11]

Table 1
Characteristics of different types of angioedema

Differential Diagnosis of AE	Clinical Characteristics	Laboratory Abnormalities	Treatment
Type I HAE	~85% of HAE cases are Type I	Low levels of complement C4 Low levels of C1-INH but it functions properly	Intravenous or subcutaneous C1-INH (recombinant or plasma-derived) Ecallantide, icatibant
Type II HAE	~15% of HAE cases are Type II Both types present with recurrent bradykinin-mediated attacks of swelling Episodes last 2–5 d Urticaria or pruritis do not occur Abdominal pain is common	Low levels of complement C4 Normal/high levels of C1-INH but it does not function properly	Danazol Lanadelumab Berotralstat Fresh frozen plasma
ACEi-induced AE	Slow onset (hours to days) of symptoms can occur any time after ACEi exposure (not just with initial dose) Up to 5 times more common in people with African descent[20] Bradykinin-mediated swelling often affects lips, tongue, face, and upper airway Abdominal pain is not common	No definitive laboratory tests	Acute airway management Discontinue ACEi Some studies suggest icatibant, others suggest antihistamines and corticosteroids
Allergic AE	Rapid onset of symptoms (within minutes to 2 h) after ingesting or contacting an allergen Histamine-mediated swelling and itching. Urticaria (hives) are extremely common Bronchospasm and hypotension are fairly common Abdominal pain and laryngeal edema are possible but not common	Normal serum complement C4 Normal C1-inhibitor function Tryptase may be elevated Treatment may include avoidance	H1 antihistamines, corticosteroids, epinephrine
Spontaneous AE	Rapid onset of symptoms (within minutes to 2 h) Histamine-mediated swelling and itching. Urticaria (hives) are often present	Normal serum complement C4 Normal C1-inhibitor function Tryptase may be elevated	H1 antihistamines, corticosteroids, and in severe cases epinephrine

Abbreviations: ACEi, angiotension converting enzyme inhibitor; AE, angioedema; HAE, hereditary angioedema.

Treatment/Management

To counteract the unregulated release of bradykinin caused by deficient or dysfunctional C1-INH, treatment of HAE includes management options for acute attacks, short-term prophylaxis (STP), and long-term prophylaxis (LTP).

Acute Attack Treatment

To deploy immediately during acute attacks, all patients with HAE should have 2 doses of on demand therapy (ODT) available. ODT focuses on reversing and preventing further angioedema. There are intravenous (IV) and SC options for ODT. The 2 IV ODT options presented are therapeutic C1-INH and fresh frozen plasma (FFP). ODT with recombinant (50 mg/kg) or plasma-derived C1-INH (20 units/kg) can be given as soon as symptoms develop.[12] It can be used in all ages and even during pregnancy and lactation. In areas where C1-INH ODT is not available due to cost, FFP can be used IV as well. FFP is not as effective as CI-INH; time-to-resolution is slower and adverse events are more frequent.[13]

The 2 SC options presented are a bradykinin-receptor antagonist called ecallantide and a kallikrein inhibitor called icatibant. Both are effective and have less clinical burden than IV therapy. Ecallantide has a 3% risk of allergic reaction and cannot be self-administered. If appropriate, a trained health-care professional can give the injection in a patient's home. Icatibant is approved only in the United States for patients aged 18 years and older. In the E.U., icatibant is approved down to 2 years of age. Because of storage ease, generic availability and injection ease, icatibant is the preferred therapy for ODT by most doctors and patients.[14]

Short-Term Prophylaxis

STP is often referred to as preprocedural; however, it can be used before any other known triggers of HAE attacks such as emotionally or physically significant events. The preferred STP is IV C1-INH an hour before the relevant surgical, medical, or dental procedure. STP is especially recommended if the procedure is adjacent to the airway (eg, molar extraction or upper endoscopy). As with acute attack treatment, if therapeutic C1-INH is unavailable, 2 units of FFP is an acceptable alternative for adolescents and adults.[15]

An alternative to C1-INH for STP is attenuated androgen. The most commonly used androgen is danazol 200 mg PO every 8 hours for 5 to 7 days before the procedure and 2 days after. Due to their short half-lives, ODT medications C1-INH, icatibant and ecallantide are not recommended for STP. In lower income areas, tranexamic acid (TXA) has been used for STP, but high-quality data are lacking to determine the efficacy of this intervention.[16]

Long-Term Prophylaxis

LTP aims to prevent attacks and reduce episode frequency. Akin to ODT, there are SC and IV therapies but unique to LTP is an oral (PO) option. LTP choices include IV C1-INH, SC C1-INH, SC lanadelumab, PO berotralstat, and PO danazol.[15] Additional PO options are currently being investigated.

IV C1-INH at 1000 units twice a week is about 50% effective in reducing attacks. Dosage can be increased to improve efficacy but this increases cost. SC C1-INH at 60 units/kg is about 85% effective and usually well tolerated.[12] Lanadelumab can be given SC every 2 or 4 weeks. At every 2 weeks, it is about 85% effective at decreasing attacks. If attacks are controlled after 6 months, a trial of dose reduction to every 4 weeks should be attempted to reduce cost.[15]

The PO LTP option, berotralstat, can cause gastrointestinal discomfort during the first few weeks and has a dose-dependent risk of QT prolongation. The significant drug burden reduction that comes from a PO option is unfortunately counterbalanced by a reduction in efficacy compared with the IV and SC options. Interestingly, some patients respond very well to berotralstat and have a greater reduction in frequency of attacks than the reported 50% decrease in episodes.

The second-line LTP options are androgens and tranexamic acid. Just as TXA is used without strong evidence for STP, physicians in lower income areas may use TXA for LTP for affordability. Danazol, as discussed with STP, is an oral, effective, and affordable option for LTP as well.[16] Danazol can cause polycythemia, hematuria, hyperlipidemia, transaminitis, and an increased risk of hepatocellular carcinoma. Use should be limited, especially in women because of masculinization. Danazol for LTP is typically used at a dose of 200 mg PO daily or less to reduce toxicity.

Additional Considerations

Beyond the biophysical manifestations of HAE, there are considerable psychosocial and financial consequences of the condition. Patients affected by HAE are often forced to miss work, school, or other social engagements due to frequent attacks. These disruptions can lead to reduction in quality of employment, education, and overall well-being. In one study of 500 patients with HAE, 42% of respondents noted symptoms of depression.[17] In another study, 39% of patients had depressive symptoms and 15% reported features of prominent anxiety.[18] As depression itself is thought to be a trigger for HAE attacks, appropriate management of depression and anxiety in patients with HAE is essential.[19]

SUMMARY

Although angioedema is commonly mediated by histamine, HAE represents a unique form of bradykinin-mediated swelling through the kinin-kallikrein cascade. To reduce morbidity and mortality, early diagnosis of HAE during attacks is extremely important. Patients with a family history of recurrent episodes of swelling without urticaria should be suspected of having HAE. Biochemical testing with complement C4 levels and C1-INH and C1-INH function can confirm the diagnosis. Once diagnosed, specific therapies can be prescribed to treat acute attacks and even prevent future attacks. All patients should be educated about the need for STP, trigger avoidance, self-treatment, LTP, and a referral to an allergy/immunology specialist.

CLINICS CARE POINTS

- HAE is a rare, inherited condition characterized by recurrent episodes of nonpruritic, nonpitting edema to the skin, intestines, and upper airway.

- HAE is commonly mistaken for other conditions such as allergic (mast cell-mediated) angioedema; however, HAE has a unique treatment approach.

- The key distinguishing aspects of HAE are an absence of wheals/urticaria, unresponsiveness to epinephrine, antihistamines, and corticosteroids, and laboratory abnormalities of C1 inhibitor quantity or function.

- The high mortality in patients with undiagnosed HAE underscores a need for broader physician awareness to identify these patients at an early age and initiate appropriate therapy.

DISCLOSURE

Dr T. Craig declares the following conflicts of interest: Research—CSL Behring, Ionis, Biocryst, Takeda, Pharvaris, BioMarin, Kalvista. Speaker—Grifols, Takeda, CSL Behring. Consultant—BioMarin, CSL Behring, Takeda, Biocryst, Spark. Drs A. Sarkar and C. Nwagwu have no conflicts to report.

REFERENCES

1. Lunn ML, Santos CB, Craig TJ. Is there a need for clinical guidelines in the United States for the diagnosis of hereditary angioedema and the screening of family members of affected patients? Ann Allergy Asthma Immunol 2010;104:211–4.
2. Bork K, Hardt J, Witzke G. Fatal laryngeal attacks and mortality in hereditary angioedema due to C1-INH deficiency. J Allergy Clin Immunol 2012;130(3):692–7.
3. Lumry WR, Settipane RA. Hereditary angioedema: Epidemiology and burden of disease. Allergy Asthma Proc 2020;41(Suppl 1):S08–13.
4. Zuraw BL. Hereditary angioedema. N Engl J Med 2008;359:1027–36.
5. Wilkerson RG, Moellman JJ. Hereditary angioedema. Emerg Med Clin North Am 2022;40(1):99–118.
6. Wu Y. Contact pathway of coagulation and inflammation. Thromb J 2015 May 6; 13:17.
7. Kashuba E, Bailey J, Allsup D, et al. The kinin-kallikrein system: physiological roles, pathophysiology and its relationship to cancer biomarkers. Biomarkers 2013;18(4):279–96.
8. Zuraw BL, Christiansen SC. HAE pathophysiology and underlying mechanisms. Clinic Rev Allerg Immunol 2016;51:216–29.
9. Bork K, Meng G, Staubach P, et al. Hereditary angioedema: new findings concerning symptoms, affected organs, and course. Am J Med 2006;119(3):267–74.
10. Henao MP, Kraschnewski JL, Kelbel T, et al. Diagnosis and screening of patients with hereditary angioedema in primary care. Ther Clin Risk Manag 2016;12: 701–11.
11. Bork K, Gül D, Hardt J, et al. Hereditary angioedema with normal C1 inhibitor: clinical symptoms and course. Am J Med 2007;120(11):987–92.
12. Bowen T, Cicardi M, Farkas H, et al. 2010 International consensus algorithm for the diagnosis, therapy and management of hereditary angioedema. All Asth Clin Immun 2010;6:24.
13. Wentzel N, Panieri A, Ayazi M, et al. Fresh frozen plasma for on-demand hereditary angioedema treatment in South Africa and Iran. World Allergy Organ J 2019; 12(9):100049.
14. Bork K, Wulff K, Witzke G, et al. Treatment for hereditary angioedema with normal C1-INH and specific mutations in the F12 gene (HAE-FXII). Allergy 2017;72(2): 320–4.
15. Banerji A, Riedl MA, Bernstein JA, et al. Effect of lanadelumab compared with placebo on prevention of hereditary angioedema attacks: a randomized clinical trial. JAMA 2018;320(20):2108–21 [published correction appears in JAMA. 2019 Apr 23;321(16):1636].
16. Caballero T. Treatment of Hereditary Angioedema. J Investig Allergol Clin Immunol 2021;31(1):1–16.
17. Lumry WR, Castaldo AJ, Vernon MK, et al. The humanistic burden of hereditary angioedema: impact on health-related quality of life, productivity, and depression. Allergy Asthma Proc 2010;31:407e414.

18. Fouche AS, Saunders EF, Craig T. Depression and anxiety in patients with hereditary angioedema. Ann Allergy Asthma Immunol 2014;112(4):371–5.
19. Bygum A, Aygören-Pürsün E, Beusterien K, et al. Burden of illness in hereditary angioedema: a conceptual model. Acta Derm Venereol 2015;95(6):706–10.
20. Brown NJ, Ray WA, Snowden M, et al. Black Americans have an increased rate of angiotensin converting enzyme inhibitor-associated angioedema. Clin Pharmacol Ther 1996;60(1):8–13.

Venom Hypersensitivity

J. Lane Wilson, MD[a],*, Bridgid Wilson, MD, PhD[b]

KEYWORDS

- Venom hypersensitivity • Anaphylaxis • Venom immunotherapy
- Stinging hymenoptera • Stinging insect • Imported fire ant • Spider bite
- Widow spider

KEY POINTS

- Stinging reactions to Hymenoptera are a common cause of local and systemic, including anaphylactic, reactions.
- Venom immunotherapy is highly effective and safe for patients with a history of a systemic reaction to Hymenoptera sting that exceeds cutaneous manifestations and who have positive venom-specific skin prick testing and/or serum-specific immunoglobulin E testing.
- Hypersensitivity to spider bite venom and scorpion sting venom is uncommon, and most local and systemic reactions to are direct effects of the venom rather than immune-mediated.

INTRODUCTION

Encounters with stinging insects, and, to a lesser extent, real or perceived encounters with stinging and biting arachnids, are a common reasons patients seek care. As the planet warms, many of these encounters will be on the rise in the United States.[1] Reactions to envenomation range from normal and localized to life-threatening anaphylaxis or direct toxicity. Envenomation from other animals, such as snakes, jellyfish, and other marine life, is less common, rarely leads to hypersensitivity reactions, and therefore is not in the scope of this article. Recognition of the spectrum of hypersensitivity reactions from envenomation from Hymenoptera and arachnids and their appropriate follow-up may prevent life-threatening reactions in the future.

HYMENOPTERA

Insects of the order Hymenoptera are a frequent cause of both local and systemic allergic reactions after stings (**Table 1**) and represent a top-two cause of anaphylaxis

---

[a] Department of Community and Family Medicine, University of Missouri Kansas City School of Medicine, University Health Lakewood Medical Center, 7900 Lee's Summit Road, Kansas City, MO 64139, USA; [b] Department of Community and Family Medicine, University Health Lakewood Medical Center, Kansas City, MO, USA
* Corresponding author.
E-mail address: lane.wilson@uhkc.org

Prim Care Clin Office Pract 50 (2023) 305–324
https://doi.org/10.1016/j.pop.2023.01.005
0095-4543/23/© 2023 Elsevier Inc. All rights reserved.

among both children and adults.[2] Most people will experience a Hymenoptera sting in their lifetime.[3] The order Hymenoptera includes the clade Anthophila (bees), family Vespidae (wasps), and family Formicidae (ants). Species and their distribution in the United States are listed in (**Table 2**). Although not exhaustive, these species make up the vast majority of Hymenoptera stings that result in hypersensitivity reactions and subsequent medical care in the United States. Africanized honeybees, vespids, and imported fire ants (IFAs) are likely to increase in range and number with climate change, and conversely, the western honeybee and bumblebees may be threatened. In total, human and stinging Hymenoptera encounters are likely to increase as the planet warms.[1]

EPIDEMIOLOGY

Approximately 40.7% of the general population has detectable immunoglobulin E (IgE) against Hymenoptera venom. Although the presence of this marker in the asymptomatic patient may predict a risk for a large local reaction (LLR), it correlates poorly with the risk for systemic reactions (SRs).[8,9] Approximately 7.5% of adults and 3.4% of children may have SRs to a Hymenoptera sting, and approximately 3.3% of Americans do.[2] Despite this widespread sensitization and nearly ubiquitous exposure over a lifetime, fatalities are rare. From 2000 to 2017, an average of 62 Americans, 80% male, die from Hymenoptera stings annually. The discrepancy in sex is thought to be due to increased exposure rather than biologic.[10] Most fatalities occur in patients without a history of SR from Hymenoptera and within 10 to 15 min of the sting.[10,11]

STINGING HYMENOPTERA
Bees

Honeybees (**Fig. 1**) and bumblebees (**Fig. 2**), family *Apidae*, are docile by nature and only sting when provoked (see **Table 1**). When honeybees sting, the stinger is left embedded, eviscerating and killing the bee in the process. The venom sac is therefore usually attached and can continue to envenomate the wound. In contrast, bumblebees do not leave behind a stinger and can therefore sting multiple times. The Africanized "killer" bee is a hybrid between the western domestic honeybee (*Apis mellifera*) and the East African lowland honeybee (*Apis mellifera scutellata*). The subspecies cannot be visually distinguished from *A mellifera* with the naked eye, and its primary difference clinically stems from its more aggressive nature, often resulting in more stings in an attack. They react to disturbances an order of magnitude faster than *A mellifera* and with more bees. Swarms have been reported to give chase to a person for up to a quarter of a mile. Although their venom is no more potent than that of *A mellifera*, the sheer number of stings delivered in attacks and aggressiveness have earned them the nickname of "killer" bees.[5,12,13]

More than 500 species of sweat bees (**Fig. 3**), family Halictidae, are known to inhabit North America. They may have similar color and banding patterns as honeybees but have a vast range of markings and coloration from black and brown to metallic greens and blues. All are small (1/4 to 3/4 inch) and docile and have earned the common name of sweat bee due to their attraction to the salts and moisture of perspiration. As such, most stings result when people swat at a female who has landed for a drink or when one is caught between skin and clothing. They do not swarm and therefore do not tend to cause large numbers of stings in a given individual.[5,14,15]

Vespids

The family Vespidae includes wasps, hornets, and yellow jackets. Paper wasps are moderately aggressive and may nest on homes, barns, sheds, fences, and playground

Table 1
Stinging Hymenoptera in the United States

	Description	Nesting	Behavior	Sting Multiple Times?	Stinger Left Embedded?	Range	Schmidt Sting Pain Index[a 4]
Clade Anthophila							
Honeybee (see **Fig. 1**)	10 to 15 mm long; red/brown with black and orange-yellow bands on the abdomen; carry pollen on legs	In caves, rock cavities, and hollow trees; usually 1 to 5 m above ground with a downward-facing entrance; up to 80,000 individuals	Docile, sting only when provoked	No	Yes	Throughout the USA	2
Bumblebee (see **Fig. 2**)	1.5 to 2.5 cm long; hairy; black with yellow or orange-yellow bands	Under vegetation, in abandoned rodent burrows, or other pre-existing cavities on or near the ground; may contain 50 to 400 members	Docile, sting only when provoked	Yes	No	Throughout the USA	1
Africanized bee (domestic and African honeybee hybrid)	Indistinguishable physically from domestic honeybee	See honeybee	Aggressive, known to swarm and give chase	No	Yes	Southwest: Louisiana, Texas, New Mexico, Arizona, California, Nevada	1

(continued on next page)

Table 1
(continued)

	Description	Nesting	Behavior	Sting Multiple Times?	Stinger Left Embedded?	Range	Schmidt Sting Pain Index[a 4]
Sweat bee (see **Fig. 3**)	Diverse size and features; 4 to 15 mm; usually brown or black, often metallic quality; may be green, blue, purple, or red and iridescent	Underground or in wood, small numbers of females may share	Docile, females sting only when provoked; known for landing on humans to obtain salts and moisture from perspiration	Can but uncommon	No	Throughout the USA	1
Family Vespidae							
Paper wasps	2 to 3 cm long and slender with narrow waist; may have red, brown, black, and/or yellow coloration	On branches, houses (particularly eaves and overhangs, attics, sheds; gray or brown umbrella-shaped nests with honeycomb-like partitions	Moderately aggressive but sting only when threatened	Yes	No	Throughout the USA	1.5
Yellow jacket (see **Fig. 4**)	10 to 15 mm in length; mostly yellow faces with black eyes, alternating black and yellow pattern on abdomen	Concealed underground; may contain up to 3,000 individuals	Nests in the ground, attracted to garbage bins and human food and drink; aggressive	Yes	Occasionally	Throughout the USA, most common in the Southeast	2

Hornets (white/bald-faced hornet and yellow hornet)	12 to 15 mm in length; black bodies and white-patterned face	In trees more than 3 but often higher than 10 to 12 feet off the ground; also may nest in attics, walls; paper-like outer shell surrounds 3 to 4 tiers of combs; may contain up to 400 individuals	Aggressively defend nests	Yes	No	Throughout the USA, most common in the Southeast	2
Family Formicidae							
Imported fire ant (red and black)	3 to 8 mm long; reddish-brown or black bodies	Dome-shaped mounts of disturbed soil; often found near sidewalks, open lawns; may contain up to 500,000 individuals	Aggressive when nest disturbed and quickly swarm; individuals sting multiple times in a radial pattern; stings are followed by local swelling and wheals within minutes and characteristic pustules within 1 to 2 days that spontaneously resolve over several days	Yes	No	Southern United States	1

a Entomologist Justin Schmidt developed a pain scale from 1 to 4 after subjecting himself to stings by a wide variety of insects.

Table 2
Hymenoptera sting reactions

	Description	Risk of Future Systemic Reaction	Acute Management	Time to Resolution	Indication for Venom-Specific IgE Testing
Local (normal)	Mild swelling, itching, burning, and erythema in small area around sting	Baseline	Often none required Topical: cold compresses, steroid creams/lotions, lidocaine Oral: antihistamines	Hours to days	No
Large local reaction (LLR)	Swellings of ≥10 cm contiguous with sting site, increases in size over 1 to 2 days	5% to 10% for any SR; <3% for severe anaphylaxis	Cold compresses, oral analgesics, nonsedating antihistamines; consider short course of oral steroids if swelling is severe or on face/neck	3 to 10 days	No
Cutaneous systemic reaction (also sometimes known as "mild anaphylaxis")	Urticaria, pruritus, flushing, or angioedema distant from sting site or generalized without other organ system symptoms	5% to 10% for any SR; <3% for more severe anaphylaxis	Nonsedating antihistamines	<24 h	Consider in some cases[a]
Anaphylaxis	Distributive shock, bronchospasm, urticarial, angioedema	30% to 60%	Intra-muscular epinephrine		Yes
Delayed hypersensitivity	Serum sickness, rhabdomyolysis, hemolytic uremic syndrome, cerebral edema, neuropathy	Undefined	Supportive, glucocorticoids	Variable, onset is 3 to 14 days after sting	Yes
Toxic/massive envenomation	Large number of stings resulting in large-dose envenomation	Undefined	Supportive	Variable	Yes (due to difficulty distinguishing from anaphylaxis)

[a] High risk of additional exposure (such as with certain occupations), high levels of anxiety regarding future reactions.[5–7]

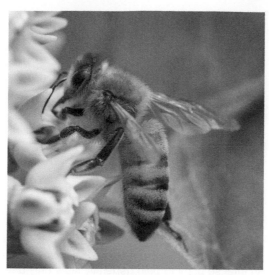

Fig. 1. Honeybee. Copyright 2016 Paula Sharp.

equipment. The honeycomb-patterned nests produced from gathered fibers mixed with their saliva have a papery texture that has resulted in the nontaxonomic term paper wasp, which mostly includes the vespid subfamily Polistinae. They are typically solitary insects, as opposed to the other clinically relevant vespids, and therefore do not swarm, making large numbers of stings uncommon.

Yellow jackets (**Fig. 4**), in contrast, are social insects and therefore can swarm when nests are disturbed, potentially resulting in many stinging injuries. They also commonly encounter people with food and drink outside, such as when picnicking, and are fairly aggressive. They represent the most common cause of SR among the Hymenoptera in the United States.[5] Hornets aggressively defend nests, often large and located in trees or shrubs, and can swarm in large numbers. They inject a higher volume of venom per sting than other Hymenoptera and do not leave a stinger.[6,16]

Imported Fire Ants

There are two species of IFAs in the United States: the red imported fire ant (RIFA), *Solenopsis invicta*, and the black imported fire ant (BIFA), *S richteri*. Both are native to South America and are considered invasive species in the United States. The RIFA, widespread among the American South and likely spreading, has been considered among the world's worst invasive species.[17] The BIFA has a much more limited geographic range that includes small areas of northwestern Mississippi, northeastern Alabama, and southern Tennessee.[18] Both species cause similar clinical manifestations.

In endemic parts of the country, RIFAs are hard to avoid, and most people suffer stings at some point. In fact, about half of people new to a RIFA endemic area experience stings within weeks of arrival.[19] Even patients who are undergoing immunotherapy continue to suffer additional stings at a similar rate to the general population.[20] Nests can be large and are typically located in open areas like fields, near sidewalks, and on playgrounds. When the nests are disturbed the ants quickly and aggressively mobilize to defend it, stinging multiple times. First, the ant anchors

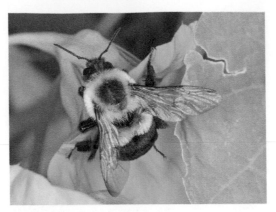

Fig. 2. Bumblebee. Copyright 2016 Paula Sharp.

to the skin with the mandibles, then uses the stinger on its abdomen to sting in an arc six to eight times. An intense burning pain generally lasts only a few minutes before subsiding. A dermal flare and wheal arises within minutes, papules develop within a few hours, and characteristic sterile pseudopustules develop at the sting sites within 1 to 2 days and resolve within 10 (**Fig. 5**).[5,6,16,18]

SHORT-TERM TREATMENT
Removal of Stinger

All stinging sites should be examined for the presence of an embedded stinger, even if the patient is able to identify the causative species, as occasionally any type of stinging Hymenoptera (with the exception of IFAs) may leave behind a stinger. In the case of honeybees and bumblebees, the venom sac is often attached. Thus, it is possible to increase venom delivery if embedded stingers are not handled carefully. A blunt-edged knife or credit card can be used to sweep across the sting site at a nearly parallel trajectory to dislodge the stinger without directing more venom into the wound. This method avoids additional envenomation and disengages the barbs of the stinger from tissue. The use of tweezers or forceps risks the introduction of additional venom and/or the breaking of the fragile stinger.[21]

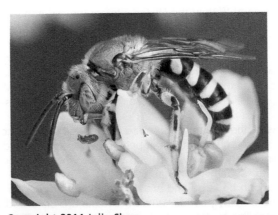

Fig. 3. Sweat bee. Copyright 2014 Julio Sharp.

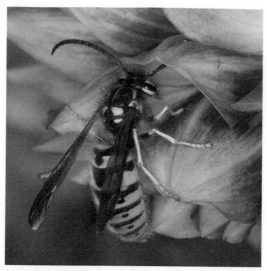

Fig. 4. Yellow jacket. Copyright 2016 Paula Sharp.

Local Reactions

Swelling, pain, pruritus, and erythema in a small area around the sting is a normal reaction and can be treated supportively. Ice or cool compresses, topical lidocaine, and topical low-to mid-potency corticosteroids may be applied.[6] Oral antihistamines are also an option, although there are likely mechanisms of pruritus resulting from Hymenoptera stings that are not histamine-mediated.[22] Large local reactions (LLRs) are similarly managed supportively; however, a short course of oral steroids may be considered in addition if symptoms are severe, worsening, or involve the head or neck (**Fig. 6**).[6]

Cutaneous Systemic Reactions

Cutaneous SRs are treated more like local reactions than anaphylactic reactions and carry a similarly low risk of a future anaphylactic reaction. Antihistamines are the

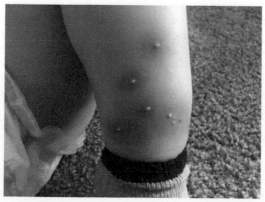

Fig. 5. Characteristic pseudopustules 24 h after RIFA stings in a toddler.

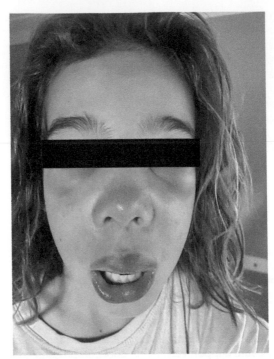

Fig. 6. Large location reaction (LLR) 48 h following bee sting (unknown species) on the lip in an 8-year-old girl.

mainstay for symptomatic urticaria which typically resolve within 24 h. Corticosteroids are not indicated given this limited time to resolution.[5,6]

Anaphylaxis

Anaphylaxis due to Hymenoptera stings is acutely managed in the same way as other etiologies of anaphylaxis. Intramuscular administration of epinephrine (0.01 mg/kg of a 1:1000 solution up to 0.3 mg in children and 0.5 mg in adults) is the only effective medical therapy and should be used first-line for anaphylaxis due to stinging Hymenoptera.[2] Multiple studies have shown underutilization of epinephrine when indicated, both in cases of anaphylaxis in general and specifically to cases caused by Hymenoptera stings.[19,23–25] Late administration of epinephrine is associated with a higher risk of mortality, and most venom-related deaths occur within 10 to 15 min of the sting.[11] Predictors of severe anaphylaxis include the absence of urticaria and angioedema, short interval onset of anaphylaxis from the time of sting, underlying systemic indolent mastocytosis (more easily measured by the surrogate basal serum tryptase level), older age, and comorbid cardiovascular disease.[26,27] Although theoretical models and early case reports had previously suggested beta-blockers and angiotensin-converting enzyme inhibitors may worsen anaphylaxis, subsequent data have not shown a significant effect or has significant limitations, and routine discontinuation is not recommended.[2,26]

Epinephrine increases systemic vascular resistance, increases heart rate, decreases bronchospasm and airway edema, and stabilizes mast cells and basophils. To maximize venous return, patients should remain in the recumbent position during resuscitation (and possibly with their legs raised), as an association with sitting up or standing during anaphylaxis and death has been observed.[28,29] About 1 in 10 cases of anaphylaxis require more than one dose of epinephrine; however, the rate in venom-induced anaphylaxis may be significantly higher.[30]

Other therapies commonly given for the treatment of anaphylaxis include non-sedating antihistamines, intravenous fluids, bronchodilators, and supplemental oxygen. Antihistamines may help with urticaria and acute pruritus, but they do not have another shown clinical role and do not prevent a biphasic reaction. Intravenous fluids are a supportive treatment to increase intravascular volume; however, epinephrine is far more important to address the etiology driving the distributive shock of anaphylaxis. Bronchodilators and supplemental oxygen are similarly supportive and adjunctive in nature to the airway effects epinephrine offers.[2,6]

Approximately 20% of patients presenting with anaphylaxis will suffer a biphasic reaction up to 72 h after the initial episode. Corticosteroids are frequently administered in an effort to prevent this sequelae; however, the evidence is now clear they are not effective and thus these agents are no longer recommended in the treatment of anaphylaxis.[2,31] Patients with severe anaphylaxis, those who require multiple doses of epinephrine, and those who have delayed treatment of anaphylaxis are at the highest risk for a biphasic reaction. These patients should be observed at least 6 h following resolution of symptoms per guideline recommendations, and others at least 1 h.[2]

Delayed Hypersensitivity Reactions

A wide variety of delayed hypersensitivity reactions have been described following Hymenoptera stings. Serum sickness-like reactions, hemolytic uremic syndrome, immune thrombocytopenic purpura, neuropathy, and other immune-mediated reactions have been documented in the weeks following stings.[32–36]

Toxic/Massive Envenomation

Toxic envenomation can result when large numbers of stings are suffered at once. Cardiovascular collapse, rhabdomyolysis, and organ failure occur not because of hypersensitivity reactions but because of direct venom effects. Liver failure, hemolysis, pancreatitis, myocardial infarction, and seizures have also been described as sequelae to massive envenomation.[16] Patients suffering from these conditions have often been stung hundreds of times, though hornets notably require fewer stings to result in organ failure as they tend to inject larger volumes of venom per sting.[16] Treatment is supportive and directed by the specific organ involvement.

LONG-TERM TREATMENT
Prevention

Any victim of Hymenoptera stinging reactions should be educated on prevention measures that include protective clothing and avoidance of nesting areas and outdoor attractants like food and garbage bins. Insect repellants are typically not effective measures to avoid stinging insects.[6]

Self-Injectable Epinephrine

Those with anaphylactic reactions should be prescribed and educated on the use of self-injectable epinephrine (SIE). For those who suffered cutaneous SR or LLR, a prescription of SIE is not required due to the low risk of subsequent anaphylaxis; however, there are circumstances in which it may be reasonable to do so. Patients with a high risk of additional exposure (such as with certain occupations) or high levels of anxiety regarding future reactions may warrant a shared decision-making conversation about carrying SIE.[5–7] Notably, carrying SIE has been shown to have negative effects on quality of life measures, particularly in patients not receiving venom immunotherapy (VIT), and thus may not achieve the goal of alleviating anxiety about future stings in these patients.[5,7]

Allergy Testing

Patients with a history of an anaphylactic reaction to Hymenoptera sting, recurrent LLRs, cutaneous SR with additional risk factors, delayed hypersensitivity reactions, toxic envenomation episodes, and those with mastocytosis (even if never had a Hymenoptera sting reaction) should be referred to an allergist for discussion about venom-specific allergy testing.[6,7] Testing should occur at least 3, and ideally after 6, weeks following the anaphylactic episode. Family history of any of these reactions is not an indication to test.

For flying Hymenoptera, skin testing is generally performed with both skin prick and intradermal testing. Serum venom-specific IgE testing is less sensitive than skin testing. Therefore, it is generally reserved for patients with negative skin but strong clinical suspicion of Hymenoptera allergy or in patients for whom skin testing is not possible (eg, severe atopic dermatitis, dermatographism, or use of antihistamine medications). Venom extracts from a yellow jacket, yellow hornet, white-faced hornet, wasp, and honeybee venoms are tested as there is significant cross-reactivity among all these species' venoms and patient identification of the offending species in the field is unreliable.[5,6] The exception to this pattern is sweat bees, which have low cross-reactivity with vespids and apidae.[14] For IFA, the whole-body extract is used for skin testing, and testing for flying Hymenoptera in patients with a history of SR to IFA stings is not necessary due to a lack of cross-reactivity.[6] Patients presenting for allergy testing are also often screened for mastocystosis using a basal serum tryptase. A disproportionate amount of patients with Hymenoptera allergy have mastocytosis and its presence informs future risk and, potentially, poorer response to VIT.[5–7]

Venom Immunotherapy

VIT is safe and extremely effective desensitization method to prevent future SRs in both children and adults who have suffered SRs and have shown sensitization. Its mechanism of action is thought to be multifactorial: inhibition of IgE-dependent reactions by IgG1/IgG4 blocking antibodies, T regulatory cells' suppression of Th2 immunity in favor of a Th1-mediated response, and other effects on cytokines, B regulatory cells, and dendritic cells.[37] The VIT number needed to treat adults and children with a history of anaphylaxis due to Hymenoptera stings and positive skin testing is approximately 2 and 6, respectively.[5] SRs are prevented at rates as high as 84% for honeybee venom, 96% for vespid venom, and 98% for IFA venom in those receiving VIT.[7] In contrast to SIE carrying, VIT is associated with reports of improved quality of life measures.[7]

LLRs and anaphylaxis are possible side effects of VIT. Anaphylaxis is uncommon and occurs in less than 5% of patients. LLRs, however, may occur in up to 50% of patients undergoing VIT. Pretreatment with H1 antihistamines reduces both the incidence and severity of this, and LLRs during VIT are not a contraindication to continuing it.[6,7] Those experiencing anaphylaxis are often able to continue VIT with dosage alterations going forward.[7]

VIT initiation protocols vary but maintenance shots are generally every 4 weeks the first year, then every 6 weeks. Generally, VIT should continue for 3 to 5 years. Long-term data on effectiveness are not available beyond 10 years, although honeybee

VIT is typically lifelong.[6,7] Despite its effectiveness, patients on maintenance dosing or completed courses of VIT, SIE should continue to be carried.[6,7]

DIPTERA

Mosquitoes, flies, and gnats make up a large number of species within the large order of 2-winged insects Diptera. The bites from these insects generally result in only small local reactions that often do not present to medical care. An important, though uncommon, exception is a hypersensitivity reaction to peptides contained within mosquito saliva termed skeeter syndrome. Within a minute of the bite a cellulitic-like reaction develops with erythema, warmth, and pruritis. Within hours, vesicles, bullae, and/or ecchymosis may occur. Because of its clinical appearance it is often mistaken for cellulitis and treated with antibiotics; however, the rapid onset and spread after mosquito bite can avoid this misdiagnosis. Severe reactions may be treated with oral corticosteroids. Allergy testing is not recommended and no specific immunotherapy is available.[38,39]

ARACHNIDS

Unlike Hymenoptera, envenomation from arachnids is unlikely to cause hypersensitivity reactions. Most envenomation accidents from spiders and scorpions result in localized and SRs that are not immune-mediated, yet can pose considerable risk depending on the degree of envenomation. Spiders and scorpions are found on all continents except Antarctica, and most do not pose a significant risk to humans.

Scorpions

Scorpions (order: Scorpione) are found in arid and desert climates with the most species diversity found in subtropical areas. Of the nearly 2000 species, only approximately 25 are potentially dangerous to humans. Species in Asia, Africa, and South America pose the greatest risk, but in North America and Mexico *Centruroides* species are venomous. Despite this, there have been no reported deaths from scorpion envenomation since the late 1960s.[40] Humans are most likely to encounter scorpions in outdoor environments, and, while not innately aggressive, envenomation accidents are most likely to occur when the scorpion feels threatened.

The vast majority of scorpion stings are "dry," meaning no or very little venom is introduced. The venom is composed of mucopolysarccharides, oligopeptides, nucleotides, and neurotoxins resulting in membrane destabilization and subsequent neuromuscular dysfunction. The most common result of a sting is localized pain and paresthesia at the sting site. Severe stings, where more venom is introduced, can result in cranial nerve and skeletal and neuromuscular dysfunction that presents as tetany, inability to control the movement of the extremities, visual changes, nystagmus, and rapid tongue movements. Other symptoms include vomiting, bronchospasm, diaphoresis, and tachycardia. Rarely cardiovascular collapse requiring inotropes can occur.[40]

Spiders

In contrast to scorpions, humans are far more likely to encounter venomous spiders (order: Araneae) given the order's ability to tolerate a wide thermal range and environmental changes, as well as good variability in feeding habits. Spiders may commonly be found in garages, storage spaces, attics, and inside homes in addition to outdoor environments. Of the more than 45,000 species of spiders only around 30 species are known to pose a significant threat to humans. Two of the best-known venomous spider species are *Latrodectus* species, most commonly known as widow spiders, and *Loxosceles* species, commonly known as recluse spiders.

Latrodectus spp
Although *Lactrodectus* species are found worldwide, approximately 44% of these species can be found in the United States.[39] Common names include black widow and button spider. *Lactrodectus* species are often identified by their dark color with red and or white markings on the dorsal and ventral aspects of the body. Only bites from females are dangerous. They show low aggression and low lethality overall. More accidents are reported in warmer months, but given that these species are commonly found in domiciles, there is a stable occurrence of accidents throughout the year.

Widow spider venom consists of proteins, peptides, and proteases with the primary toxin being alpha-latrotoxin. The alpha-latrotoxin binds irreversibly to receptors on presynaptic neurons causing the release of neurotransmitters. Bites are characterized by quick and severe burning pain at the envenomation site. Generalized myalgia and muscle spasms may occur in a contiguous spread and intensify over time. Other symptoms associated with bites include rhinitis, salivation, anxiety, blepharitis, and masseter trismus. Rarely, rhabdomyolysis and oliguria with acute kidney injury (AKI) may occur. Some data support that the mechanism behind AKI is independent of rhabdomyolysis.[41,42]

Loxoceles spp
Similar to *Lactrodectus* species, *Loxoceles* species show a worldwide distribution. Common names for these species include brown recluse, brown spider, fiddle-back spider, violin spiders, and reapers. These spiders are nocturnal and nonaggressive, with most accidents occurring when a human accidentally presses up against the spider, such as in bedding or in clothing.

Recluse spider bites may be more difficult to identify than a widow spider bite due to the initial bite often being painless. Consequently, symptoms may not begin to be recognized until 2 to 8 h later. Active components of recluse venom include proteases that degrade components of the extracellular matrix, as well as sphingomyelinase D that can cause toxin-mediated hemolysis and complement-mediated erythrocyte destruction.[43] Sequelae of recluse spider bites can be categorized into cutaneous loxoscelism (CL) and cutaneous-visceral loxoscelism (CVL).[43,44] CL is characterized by erythema with a central ulceration and necrosis, which often progresses to eschar with well-delineated borders. Other symptoms such as malaise, low-grade fever, and nausea may also occur. Typically the cutaneous findings do not peak until 7 to 14 days after the bite. CVL has the same cutaneous findings as CL with the addition of multiple systemic events including complement-mediated hemolysis, cytokine activation resulting in possible shock, acute tubular necrosis, and renal insufficiency, and DIC.[44] Of note CVL may have insidious development over 7 to 14 days, making anticipatory guidance critically important in acute settings after the initial bite.

Epidemiology and Diagnosis
The vast majority of spider and scorpion accidents are mild with only local reactions, so there is likely a significant amount of underreporting as most envenomation accidents can be and are treated at home with supportive care only. Additionally, envenomation events, particularly by spiders, are difficult to confirm as the actual event is often unwitnessed and patients may inappropriately assume other dermatologic conditions, such as abscesses, are from a spider bite. In addition to unwitnessed events,

another complicating factor regarding the epidemiology of envenomation events is a relatively wide range of reaction. Depending on the degree of envenomation, reactions can range from localized pain and erythema to systemic effects, shock, and death. It is feasible that some more severe cases may be underrepresented as an onset to cardiovascular collapse or acute renal impairment may present several days after the accident leading to misdiagnosis of the etiology. In one study looking at a 4-year period of nearly 1.2 million Emergency Department visits for animal bites and stings, an estimated 120,572 visits were for spider bites but only 2.7% of those visits were associated with venomous spiders. Scorpion stings comprised almost 8,000 visits (~6%).[45]

As previously mentioned many patients may assume they have incurred a spider bite when in reality their "bite" is actually a diagnosis from an impressively long list of conditions that may masquerade as a spider bite. Complicating matters further is the natural history of brown recluse bites, which often do not peak with ulceration more than 7 days after the accident. Consequently, a useful mnemonic—NOT RECLUSE—has been described by Stoecker and colleagues[46] that describes features that are not common to recluse spider bites that will help physicians and providers eliminate recluse spider bites from their differential diagnosis. This mnemonic can be found in **Table 3**.

TREATMENT
Scorpion Sting

As mentioned previously most scorpion stings are dry, meaning little to no venom is transmitted. Treatment includes general cleansing of the area, and analgesia with medications such as nonsteroidal anti-inflammatory drug or acetaminophen. In patients experiencing more systemic symptoms such as agitation and muscle spasticity benzodiazepines can be used. Gastrointestinal manifestations can be treated with medications such as antiemetics.[40,47] Some patients may experience hypertension in less severe reactions and anti-hypertensive medications such as nifedipine, prazosin, and beta-blockers can be considered.[47] Given that the amount of venom introduced by the scorpion is variable it is reasonable to observe patients for at least 4 h before discharge to ensure they do not develop more serious signs of SR.[40] For those patients experiencing more severe reactions, including cardiovascular collapse, and pulmonary distress such as pulmonary edema, hyperthermia, and rhabdomyolysis, transfer to an intensive care setting should be considered. Although treatment measures are predominantly still supportive, the availability of inotropes and vasopressors as well as advanced airway resources is critical. Children appear to be at greater risk for more severe complications.

Treatment is available for scorpion stings in the form of IV F(ab')2 equine antivenom. There have been no reported cases of anaphylaxis caused by the antivenom, though serum sickness has been reported.[40] Some controversy exists regarding the use of scorpion antivenom. The onset of action of scorpion venom is very quick due to the components having the low molecular weight and consequently faster absorption into circulation into subcutaneous tissue.[47] Administration of antivenom is most effective within 4 h of the sting, which may be challenging depending on when the patient is able to present to care and delay in treatment due to wait times. Additionally, newer formulations of the antivenom are exceedingly expensive and may not always be available in hospitals in endemic areas.[40] Nevertheless, in severe cases refractory to supportive care antivenom should be considered.

Widow Spider Bite

Widow spider bites are most commonly treated with supportive care that focuses on analgesia with NSAIDs and opioids and the treatment of muscle spasms with

Table 3
NOT RECLUSE mnemonic

Letter	Characteristic	Description
N	Numerous	Numerous lesions are atypical for recluse spider bites. If more than one lesion is present consider an alternative diagnosis.
O	Occurrence	Typical recluse bites occur when the spider has been disturbed such as when going through boxes in an attic or when a human comes in contact with bedding the spider may have been in.
T	Timing	Though recluse bites can occur year-round the most active months in North America are April-October.
R	Red	Owing to local destruction of vasculature from the venom-causing ischemia, the central aspect of recluse bites tends to be white or pale. If the center of the lesion is erythematous expand the differential diagnosis.
E	Elevated	Recluse spider bites are typically flat or sunken. Elevated lesions suggest an alternative diagnosis.
C	Chronic	Though dermonecrosis from recluse bites can be impressive, lesions are typically healed within 3 months. If the lesions are persisting beyond 3 months consider an alternative diagnosis.
L	Large	It is exceedingly uncommon for recluse bites to expand beyond 10 cm in diameter.
U	Ulcerates too early	Typical ulceration for recluse bites occurs at least 7 days after the initial bite.
S	Swollen	Recluse spider bites do not typically cause impressive swelling. The exception to this are bites on the neck and face.
E	Exudate	Recluse spider bites are not exudative. If the lesion is purulent consider an alternative diagnosis.

If 2 or More NOT RECLUSE Criteria Are Present an Alternative Diagnosis is Strongly Suggested.[44]

benzodiazepines. Historically calcium gluconate and methocarbamol have been used for symptom reduction, though these have fallen out of favor due to lack of efficacy.[41] For more severe cases that are complicated by pulmonary edema, cardiac failure, and renal impairment maintaining an appropriate airway and supportive care is the mainstay of treatment. An antivenom exists for widow spider bites that is both very affordable, has an excellent reduction in symptoms, and is effective against all *Latrodectus* species; however, the antivenom is only given in less than 4% of confirmed cases. This surprising lack of use of antivenom is likely due to concerns about anaphylaxis. Rare cases of anaphylaxis and 2 reported cases of fatalities from the antivenom have been reported, though in both fatalities the patients had an underlying complication of asthma. Consequently if considering using *Latrodectus* antivenom a thorough medical history for asthma and atopy should be performed.[41,44]

Recluse Spider Bite

CL follows a typical course that starts with a pale center with an erythematous border around the initial bite secondary to vasoconstriction. Over the course of the next 7 to 14 days, it is not uncommon for a central blister to form and ultimately ulcerate with a blue or violet sunken center.[43] Formation of an eschar with eventual skin sloughing follows with healing by secondary intention. It is important to counsel patients on the typical progression of the lesion and provide adequate anticipatory guidance regarding complications of healing, such as secondary cellulitis. Without secondary complications, recluse spider bites only require general cleansing and local wound care. There was a historic practice of using topical dapsone to help with healing though this is not only unnecessary but reports of anaphylaxis to dapsone have been reported.[43] Additionally, surgical debridement of eschar is contraindicated as this may increase inflammatory response and negatively affect healing.[43,44] CVL is treated primarily by supportive care for the sequelae of hemolysis, renal impairment, and cardiovascular collapse. An antivenom does exist for *Loxosceles* species, though unlike *Latrodectus* antivenom it is unlikely to work for all species, and it is not effective against dermonecrosis. The antivenom may be used for the treatment and prevention of CVL.[44]

As with other spider and scorpion bites pediatric patients are at higher risk for severe complications. Given that the onset of hemolysis and renal failure may not occur until 7 to 14 days after the initial bite, it is critical to caution patients and caregivers to be aware of this complication.[43]

SUMMARY

Patients frequently encounter stinging Hymenoptera and have high rates of sensitization and risk for SRs to stings. Anaphylactic reactions should be treated with intramuscular epinephrine according to evidence-based anaphylaxis guidelines and subsequently referred for venom-specific IgE testing. Patients with positive skin prick testing who have a history of SR that exceeds cutaneous symptoms should be offered VIT, which is highly effective and safe. Arachnids are less likely to cause hypersensitivity reactions and more likely to result in symptoms directly from venom toxicity. Familiarity with the spectrum of reactions to Hymenoptera and arachnid stings and bites can reduce unnecessary testing and treatment as well as provide life-saving interventions for those at high risk.

CLINICS CARE POINTS

- Local and cutaneous systemic reactions to Hymenoptera stings should be treated supportively.

- Anaphylaxis due to Hymenoptera envenomation should be treated acutely with intramuscular epinephrine, and long-term, patients should be counseled on prevention strategies, prescribed self-injectable epinephrine, and referred for allergy testing and venom immunotherapy counseling.

- Venom immunotherapy is highly effective and safe and should be continued for at least 3 to 5 years in patients with a history of systemic reactions to Hymenoptera venom beyond cutaneous symptoms and positive venom-specific skin prick testing and/or serum-specific immunoglobulin E testing; treatment of honeybee allergy with venom immunotherapy can be lifelong

- Scorpion antivenom is expensive, has limited availability, and should be ideally administered within 4 h of presentation in those with severe symptoms

- Widow antivenom is highly effective but may rarely cause life-threatening anaphylaxis, particularly in patients with a history of asthma

- The NOT RECLUSE mnemonic may help clinicians who are considering recluse bite on the differential to focus on alternative diagnoses

DISCLOSURE

The authors have nothing to disclose.

REFERENCES

1. Demain JG. Insect migration and changes in venom allergy due to climate change. Immunol Allergy Clin N Am 2021;41(1):85–95.
2. Shaker MS, Wallace DV, Golden DBK, et al. Anaphylaxis-a 2020 practice parameter update, systematic review, and Grading of Recommendations, Assessment, Development and Evaluation (GRADE) analysis. J Allergy Clin Immunol 2020;145: 1082.
3. Antonicelli L, Bilò MB, Bonifazi F. Epidemiology of hymenoptera allergy. Curr Opin Allergy Clin Immunol 2002;2(4):341–6.
4. The Schmidt sting pain index, Available at: https://www.nhm.ac.uk/scroller-schmidt-painscale/#intro. Accessed August 3, 2022.
5. Ochfeld EN, Greenberger PA. Stinging insect allergy and venom immunotherapy. Allergy Asthma Proc 2019;40(6):372–5.
6. Abrams EM, Golden DBK. Approach to Patients with Stinging Insect Allergy. Med Clin North Am 2020;104(1):129–43.
7. Sturm GJ, Varga EM, Roberts G, et al. EAACI guidelines on allergen immunotherapy: Hymenoptera venom allergy. Allergy 2018;73(4):744–64.
8. Sturm GJ, Kranzelbinder B, Schuster C, et al. Sensitization to Hymenoptera venoms is common, but systemic sting reactions are rare. J Allergy Clin Immunol 2014;133(6):1635–16343.e1.
9. Sturm GJ, Schuster C, Kranzelbinder B, et al. Asymptomatic sensitization to hymenoptera venom is related to total immunoglobulin E levels. Int Arch Allergy Immunol 2009;148(3):261–4.
10. QuickStats. Number of Deaths from Hornet, Wasp, and Bee Stings, Among Males and Females — National Vital Statistics System, United States, 2000–2017. MMWR Morb Mortal Wkly Rep 2019;68:649.
11. Pumphrey RS. Fatal anaphylaxis in the UK, 1992-2001. Novartis Found Symp 2004;257:116–28 [discussion: 128-32, 157-60, 276-128].
12. Ellis, Jamie (January 2008). "Africanized honey bee - Apis mellifera scutellata Lepeletier". University of Florida Entomology and Nematology Department, Available at: https://entnemdept.ufl.edu/creatures/misc/bees/ahb.htm. Accessed August 3, 2022.
13. Africanized Bees. Information Sheet Number45. Smithsonian Institute BugInfo, Available at: https://www.si.edu/spotlight/buginfo/killbee. Accessed August 3, 2022.
14. Pence HL, White AF, Cost K, et al. Evaluation of severe reactions to sweat bee stings. Ann Allergy 1991;66(5):399–404.
15. Halictid Bees (Sweat Bees) | Missouri Department of Conservation, Available at: https://mdc.mo.gov/discover-nature/field-guide/halictid-bees-sweat-bees. Accessed August 3, 2022.
16. Schmidt JO. Clinical consequences of toxic envenomations by Hymenoptera. Toxicon 2018;150:96–104.
17. Global Invasive Species Database, 2022, Available at: http://www.iucngisd.org/gisd/100_worst.php on 15-08-2022. Accessed August 3, 2022.
18. Kruse B., Anderson J. and Simon L.V., Fire Ant Bites, In: StatPearls [Internet]. Treasure Island (FL), 2022, StatPearls Publishing,Treasure Island (FL).

19. Szari SM, Adams KE, Quinn JM, et al. Characteristics of venom allergy at initial evaluation: Is fire ant hypersensitivity similar to flying Hymenoptera? Ann Allergy Asthma Immunol 2019;123(6):590–4.
20. Letz AG, Quinn JM. Frequency of imported fire ant stings in patients receiving immunotherapy. Ann Allergy Asthma Immunol 2009;102(4):303–7.
21. Steen CJ, Janniger CK, Schutzer SE, et al. Insect sting reactions to bees, wasps, and ants. Int J Dermatol 2005;44(2):91–4.
22. Cerpes U, Repelnig ML, Legat FJ. Itch in Hymenoptera Sting Reactions. Front Allergy 2021;2:727776.
23. Prince BT, Mikhail I, Stukus DR. Underuse of epinephrine for the treatment of anaphylaxis: missed opportunities. Journal of Asthma and Allergy 2018;11:143.
24. Robinson M, Greenhawt M, Stukus DR. Factors associated with epinephrine administration for anaphylaxis in children before arrival to the emergency department. Annals of Allergy, Asthma & Immunology 2017;119(2):164–9.
25. Clark S, Boggs KM, Balekian DS, et al, MARC-38 Investigators. Changes in emergency department concordance with guidelines for the management of stinging insect-induced anaphylaxis: 1999-2001 vs 2013-2015. Ann Allergy Asthma Immunol 2018;120(4):419–23.
26. Stoevesandt J, Sturm GJ, Bonadonna P, et al. Risk factors and indicators of severe systemic insect sting reactions. Allergy 2020;75(3):535–45.
27. Chapsa M, Roensch H, Langner M, et al. Predictors of severe anaphylaxis in hymenoptera venom allergy: the importance of absence of urticaria and angioedema. Ann Allergy Asthma Immunol 2020;125(1):72–7.
28. Pumphrey RS. Fatal posture in anaphylactic shock. J Allergy Clin Immunol 2003;112(2):451–2.
29. Boulain T, Achard JM, Teboul JL, et al. Changes in BP induced by passive leg raising predict response to fluid loading in critically ill patients. Chest 2002;121(4):1245–52.
30. Patel N, Chong KW, Yip AYG, et al. Use of multiple epinephrine doses in anaphylaxis: a systematic review and meta-analysis. J Allergy Clin Immunol 2021;148(5):1307–15.
31. Alqurashi W, Ellis AK. Do corticosteroids prevent biphasic anaphylaxis? J Allergy Clin Immunol Pract 2017;5(5):1194–205.
32. Reisman RE, Livingston A. Late-onset allergic reactions, including serum sickness, after insect stings. J Allergy Clin Immunol 1989;84(3):331–7.
33. Lee YC, Wang JS, Shiang JC, et al. Haemolytic uremic syndrome following fire ant bites. BMC Nephrol 2014;15:5.
34. Koya S, Crenshaw D, Agarwal A. Rhabdomyolysis and acute renal failure after fire ant bites. J Gen Intern Med 2007;22:145–7.
35. Akbayram S, Akgun C, Dogan M, et al. Acute ITP due to insect bite: report of 2 cases. Clin Appl Thromb Hemost 2011;17(4):408–9.
36. Kutlu A, Aydin E, Goker K, et al. Cold-induced urticaria with systemic reactions after hymenoptera sting lasting for 10 years. Allergol Immunopathol (Madr) 2013;41(4):283–4.
37. Sahiner UM, Durham SR. Hymenoptera venom allergy: how does venom immunotherapy prevent anaphylaxis from bee and wasp stings? Front Immunol 2019;10:1959.
38. Simons FE, Peng Z. Skeeter syndrome. J Allergy Clin Immunol 1999;104(3 Pt 1):705–7.
39. Singh S, Mann BK. Insect bite reactions. Indian J Dermatol Venereol Leprol 2013;79(2):151–64.

40. Shamoon Z, Peterfy RJ, Hammoud S, et al. Scorpion toxicity. In: StatPearls [internet]. Treasure Island (FL): StatPearls Publishing; 2022.
41. Caruso MB, Lauria PSS, de Souza CMV, et al. Widow spiders in the New World: a review on Latrodectus Walckenaer, 1805 (Theridiidae) and latrodectism in the Americas. J Venom Anim Toxins Incl Trop Dis 2021;27:e20210011.
42. Williams M, Anderson J, Nappe TM. Black widow spider toxicity. In: StatPearls [internet]. Treasure island (FL): StatPearls Publishing; 2021. 2022.
43. Anoka IA, Robb EL, Baker MB. Brown recluse spider toxicity. In: StatPearls [internet]. Treasure island (FL): StatPearls Publishing; 2022.
44. Lopes PH, Squaiella-Baptistão CC, Marques MOT, et al. Clinical aspects, diagnosis and management of Loxosceles spider envenomation: literature and case review. Arch Toxicol 2020;94(5):1461–77.
45. Hareza D, Langley R, Haskell MG, et al. National Estimates of Noncanine Bite and Sting Injuries Treated in US Hospital Emergency Departments, 2011-2015. South Med J 2020;113(5):232–9.
46. Stoecker WV, Vetter RS, Dyer JA. NOT RECLUSE-A mnemonic device to avoid false diagnoses of brown recluse spider Bites. JAMA Dermatol 2017;153(5):377–8.
47. Abroug F, Ouanes-Besbes L, Tilouche N, et al. Scorpion envenomation: state of the art. Intensive Care Med 2020;46(3):401–10.

Moving?

Make sure your subscription moves with you!

To notify us of your new address, find your **Clinics Account Number** (located on your mailing label above your name), and contact customer service at:

Email: journalscustomerservice-usa@elsevier.com

800-654-2452 (subscribers in the U.S. & Canada)
314-447-8871 (subscribers outside of the U.S. & Canada)

Fax number: 314-447-8029

Elsevier Health Sciences Division
Subscription Customer Service
3251 Riverport Lane
Maryland Heights, MO 63043

*To ensure uninterrupted delivery of your subscription, please notify us at least 4 weeks in advance of move.

Printed and bound by CPI Group (UK) Ltd, Croydon, CR0 4YY

03/10/2024

01040471-0015